RED TENTS

Unravelling Our Past
and
Weaving a Shared Future

Mary Ann Clements and Aisha Hannibal

WOMANCRAFT PUBLISHING

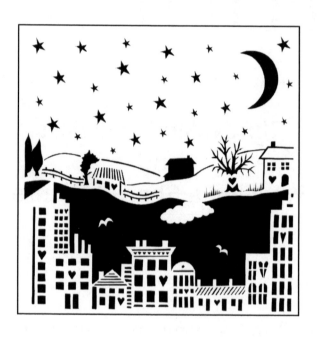

PRAISE FOR RED TENTS

This book is a bold and courageous antidote to racism, oppression and exclusion. The authors offer a step by step guide to creating liberatory Red Tent spaces where women share collective leadership, listen deeply to one another without trying to fix anything, and inclusion is a central pillar holding up the Tent. The reflective questions peppered through the book encourage a personal journey for the reader. I highly recommend this book for any woman wanting to set up or participate in a Red Tent.

Nicola Kurk, Shadow Work trainer, facilitator and coach

A must-read for women yearning to create Red Tent sisterhood. This book captures the magic of the global Red Tent movement and provides new insight into how to celebrate and honour what it means to be a woman.

Isadora Leidenfrost, PhD, Red Tent movie filmmaker *Things We Don't Talk About* and author *The Red Tent Movement: A Historical Perspective*

Brilliant. Brilliant. Brilliant. This book is so important in opening up vital conversations for those facilitating spaces for women – it feels like absolute gold dust. What is explored here is what I feel has been missing from the core values of many groups within the Red Tent movement and women's sacred circles. For those striving for more inclusive spaces, it is long overdue. I am very grateful to the writers for putting what many of us have been thinking and feeling into this very clear and well-written book. I will be buying copies for everyone I know and recommending it far and wide. Thank you.

Clare Jasmine Beloved, artist, poet, irreverent Liverpool creatrix, creative activist, circle sista, sharing the medicine in our stories and finding the magic in the margin

In this fast-moving and ever-changing world, the need for Red Tent spaces is bigger than ever. With this powerful, and at times challenging, book, Mary Ann and Aisha offer a guide to how the Red Tents of now and the future can unpick old ideas and offer brave, intersectional spaces where all voices can be heard. Whether you're new to the ways of the Red Tent or are an experienced circle leader, this visionary book is much-needed and offers necessary input from a range of experiences about how the Red Tent has the potential to co-create healing and learning communities for the benefit of all.

Awen Clement, founder of The Earth House

Refreshing, renewing, restorative and indeed, revolutionary, this book nourishes a community-based approach to Red Tents that is both anti-oppressive and expansive, guiding you into the terrain of the liberatory while simultaneously honouring the messy, embodied complexity of doing this world-changing work. This book is a good addition to the resource library of the global Red Tent movement as a whole.

Molly Remer, author of *Womanrunes*, rural Red Tent Circle priestess, Red Tent Initiation program creator, creatrix and circle-tender of Brigid's Grove

This book is a radical manifesto. It is an honest and practical manual, both challenging and reassuring by turns. Draw the curtains, pull up a comfy chair and settle down to listen to this collective weave of many voices, including your own, as you answer the many thoughtful questions it contains. Find out what being in a Red Tent could mean for you. A wise guide to making change, one rest at a time.

Liz Rothschild, author of *Outside the Box – Everyday Stories of Death, Bereavement and Life*, actor, funeral celebrant and founder of Westmill Woodland Burial Ground

Red Tents is a practical and deeply insightful invitation to firstly look at how you are nourished within your own inner world, and then to consider how you may work in collaboration with others to co-create Red Tent spaces that are truly welcoming and accessible to all women who may feel drawn to be held in the deeply calm, inclusive and courageous space Red Tents have the potential to be. An invaluable resource for everyone creating and holding safe spaces for women's authentic sharing, showing up and connection.

Clare Cooper, author of *Milestones of Motherhood*

I appreciate this very thorough examination of the many issues involved with hosting Red Tents, including cultural appropriation, gender issues, white woman spirituality and more. Much food for thought is generated by the many lessons the authors have learned to help those who have not had the experience of forming a Red Tent. Mary Ann and Aisha put deep consideration into how to bring women together for connection, inspiration and healing. And then they went back, amidst the Covid-19 pandemic, to include virtual Red Tents and how this vital work can continue in today's current environment. They've created an essential resource for those hosting Red Tents and for those who wish to do so.

Caryn MacGrandle, creator of The Divine Feminine app

Published by Womancraft Publishing, 2021
womancraftpublishing.com

ISBN 978-1-910559-57-4
Red Tents is also available in ebook format: ISBN 978-1-910559-56-7

Cover image © Leigh Millar
Design and typesetting: lucentword.com
Candles: Pular/Shutterstock.com

Womancraft Publishing is committed to sharing powerful new women's voices, through a collaborative publishing process. We are proud to midwife this work, however the story, the experiences and the words are the authors' alone. A percentage of Womancraft Publishing profits are invested back into the environment reforesting the tropics (via TreeSisters) and forward into the community.

Printed in Ireland by Carraig Print Litho Press, Cork.

For all those who have come before us, our ancestors, all the mothers, grandmothers, great-grandmothers, the elders, and the wisdom they held and passed on.

For all those who will read this book: those in our lives, women throughout the world who contribute to the collective consciousness of the many facets of 'woman' and to much-needed change in our world at this time.

For all those yet to come, yet to be born, yet to bring their wisdom and their gifts to share, who will continue the future line of women.

CONTENTS

FOREWORD
by ALisa Starkweather

As well as being the founder of the Red Tent Temple Movement I co-founded other initiatives, one of which was Women in Power in the UK. This is where I met and formed a deep and lasting bond with the authors of *Red Tents: Unravelling Our Past and Weaving a Shared Future*, Mary Ann Clements and Aisha Hannibal. From our many years together in a community which values extraordinary transformational work of facing our darkest shadows, these are women who can be trusted. Quite different from the Red Tent Temple Movement, Women in Power is a more radical body of work where women confront internal hatred from patriarchy and rewire the perpetrator-victim cycles embedded in our own trauma histories and nervous systems. Together we have witnessed first-hand the courage it requires for people to live the story of disrupting harmful ancestral lineage patterns and what it means to be held through rage and grief as the most traumatic of our wounds surface to be healed.

These authors know how to hold deep containers for the suffering of humanity's heart-break and also what supports healthy restorative relationships. They include how to make agreements, go with the flow, respect where people are at, and how to be a part of the most important social justice work of our time with facing not only patriarchy but also white supremacy embedded in our leadership, our institutions and even sometimes our most heartfelt intentions.

More than a concept, the Red Tent is a practice ground for us to learn how to get along. Our lives and communities are facing vast changes and we need tools and skills to support our ability to adapt most especially in times of crisis. Being part of Red Tent communities for years is how the authors gathered important lessons that make them the right guides for teaching people how to use them. What they offer here is not an ideology but a repertoire of skills and tools for healing.

Red Tents: Unravelling Our Past and Weaving a Shared Future contains many narratives and points of view and this includes the shifts necessary for the Red Tent movement to survive from where we first originated to what is needed now as we deepen. As truth-tellers and women who know how to be vulnerable and present, Aisha and Mary Ann amplify collective voices. Amidst our present global cultural landscapes, we see the importance and the challenge of holding containers where it is all here – women's empowerment, racial justice work, transgender politics, non-binary gender inclusion and a whole lot of ideas of what the Red Tent is, ought to be, could be, or never will be. We get to choose how we live the story.

Once I heard an elder say wisely, "Be careful how you tell the story, because how you tell the story can become the story." What will be our story to tell of the Red Tents? To delve requires openness and curiosity to the many conversations that are needed at this time for humanity's healing. How do we make this a safe and brave container that can nourish our souls, hold our hearts and expand our abilities to embrace respectfully the many stories and concerns? How do we invite those who participate to feel seen, heard and held? It will take labour, thoughtfulness, tolerance and a commitment to outcome.

A Red Tent will be different each and every time you choose to enter or choose to hold this space for yourself and others. Take a moment at the threshold of this book to ask: what has brought you to the door of the Red Tent? What is your deep longing that you are hoping can meet you on these pages?

Wherever we call home together, may we continue to foster empathy, connection, equity and healing for all. May we take the risks required to tell a new story together – one that brings us more alive and able to count on one another as siblings.

Respectfully,

ALisa Starkweather (pronouns she/her/hers)

AUTHORS' INTRODUCTION

The fire is on and the tea is brewing. The two of us are sitting together scribbling our ideas and talking passionately about the Red Tent Directory, a website that could connect women to one another and to their Red Tents.

It is sometime in 2012 and we have never worked together before, but we share enthusiasm for the idea of connecting Red Tents and helping women find them. We are deeply committed to enabling more women to access Red Tents: helping make them more open and findable, and also to them welcoming a more diverse range of women.

As we begin to connect Red Tents through our online listing site, people start to ask us for support with running them. Over time we see some patterns in what works well and the things that seem to cause challenges. Often, we help people holding Red Tents understand that if it isn't easy it doesn't mean it is wrong, that when things feel tricky it is often where the work deepens, connections grow, new ways of doing something are revealed.

After six years of running the Directory and reflecting on what we heard from an ever-growing community, we decided to write this book. Our idea was to interview women who ran and attended Red Tents and to share their stories, documenting what Red Tents are like and what they mean to the women who attend them. We thought that their stories would come together to create a guide: a way to navigate starting and running a Red Tent, facing the challenges that come up, strengthening the community and, where necessary, also letting Red Tents close.

We thought that a book that documented these stories would be another mechanism, beyond the Directory, to share the idea of Red Tents with more people.

We wrote the first draft of this book in 2019. Part of the process involved interviewing seventy-three different women and genderqueer people who run or are involved in Red Tents. We asked them all kinds of questions and found a lot to celebrate. We heard a collective vision of holding community, the depth of learning that was taking place and the gifts that rippled out far beyond the Red Tent itself in women's lives.

But we were also struck by how few Red Tents had thought about inclusion beyond the often unspoken assumption that they would figure out and adapt to women's diverse needs when, and if, they happened to present themselves. Very few had thought intentionally about including people by design and how it might affect the ways in which they promoted, held, and supported their Red Tent spaces and community.

Based on these conversations, we wrote sections in that initial draft of this book that talked about how to make your Red Tent better-equipped for racial diversity, more inclusive for trans women, more accessible for those with disabilities and how to think about money and access amongst other things.

But we knew that our writing process wasn't quite done, some things were still missing. And, in particular, that the parts of the book in which we had tried to deal with issues of access and equity were not yet what we wanted them to be.

And then 2020 happened.

We entered a global pandemic and Covid-19 took Red Tents online or into a temporary pause. Red Tents were suddenly unable to meet and had to experiment, often for the first time, with going online and this presented challenges as well as opportunities for accessibility. Lockdown provided an opportunity to write, read, think and reflect which led to deep conversations with each other and reaching out to more women in our communities and network.

Grief and anger about the murders of Black people and, in particular of, Breonna Taylor in Kentucky, Tony McDade in Florida, Ahmaud Arbery in Georgia and George Floyd in Minnesota magnified a collective movement for change, Black Lives Matter, which is led by Black, queer women in the United States. Protests and demands for justice rooted in centuries of genocide, slavery and colonisation, began to open up a deeper conversation in many parts of the world about the realities of racism in our wider cultures that was long, long overdue.

It is through this time that our conviction has grown that Red Tents can become more liberatory spaces. We know that any attempt to avoid the realities of injustice risks perpetuating it. And so, we deeply believe that we have to be asking the questions, immersing ourselves in the enquiry and committing to the practice of building spaces that feel different.

As we adapt to change forced by a crisis of health, climate, inequality and systemic injustice we have multiple opportunities to reflect on what the world is calling for right now and how we can respond. We think the practice and ritual of Red Tents can be part of imagining spaces in our lives that help us to understand together what is possible in a world that will never be the same, that will never get back to 'normal'.

We stand for creating Red Tents collectively, spaces where we practice leading together, being together, imagining together. Spaces where we bring ritual, respect and honesty to our everyday lives. Spaces where care becomes a blueprint between us. Spaces where we can engage together in the long-term work of unpicking oppressive systems.

We think that in order to make them spaces where we can think about how to heal from oppression, they also need to be places where we are comfortable with not knowing all the answers, where we can make mistakes and in which we can be active in unravelling the threads that make us feel divided in the first place. We hope that the content of this book sparks ideas to ignite conversation and reflection in your Red Tent.

As you'll read in the pages of this book, Red Tents can look different in different places. We don't think there is only one way to run one and we hope that what we offer here will feel flexible. By all means, take what you like and make it your own and appropriate to your community. You don't even have to call it a Red Tent.

For us, the essence of Red Tents is a way of connecting to one another, of taking space out of our busy lives, of hearing without needing to fix one another and of building connections that are liberatory.

You could think of Red Tents as a collective practice of care that you can co-create anywhere, that provides one small way to help contribute to calling into being a fairer and more just world. This is a lifetime's journey, a long-term practice.

We invite you towards deepening what Red Tents can offer. We are with you in every moment of indecision, doubt and delight. In fact, we can't do this without you.

PART ONE

VOICES FROM THE RED TENT

There is a sign on the entry door welcoming me in… I make my way upstairs, take off my shoes and add them to the pile. Inside I can hear the sounds of women laughing and chatting. I enter the room and join the circle absorbing it all until it is my turn to speak. Women of all ages relax together as they listen to one another.

Steph

I stand barefoot in my garden, deepening my breath, preparing for our online Red Tent. Staying connected, I move into my office and join the Zoom call, smiling as the faces of the women begin to pop up on the screen. Here we are. We take a few breaths together before anyone starts talking, before reminding women that this is their time, our time. Coming more and more into presence feels like the perfect introduction to each woman sharing where she is now, in this moment.

Debbie

In the studio next to the co-working desks, a circle of women gather on velvet cushions. In the middle of the circle is a centrepiece with flowers, seashells and river stones. It holds candles, one for each woman, which she lights to open the circle. The women range in age from seventeen to seventy. There are women who know they need this, and women who seem surprised to find themselves doing 'this kind of thing'.

Emily

We are sitting in a yurt in a field on the edge of a beautiful wood, which slopes down towards the River Thames. The yurt is used for all sorts of purposes, so we bring cushions and decorations with us. The wood stove is the first thing that I attend to as I arrive to set up the Red Tent, followed by turning on the hot water urn. I set up the centre-piece with a round red cloth that I made especially with seasonal flowers to decorate it.

Tessa

Excited giggles, shy happy smiles, hearty welcoming of mums and their daughters as they bustle in stealing time out of a busy weekend to drop into this collective space. Each landing their baskets and boxes of baked and bought food offerings in the kitchen and craft on the shared table. Mums hover over, enabling young shaky hands to light the opening candle. Everyone has a chance to bring their voice into the circle, birthdays and achievements are celebrated, struggles acknowledged, and we reflect on what we love about ourselves and one another.

Mads

[A Red Tent] is a space for silence and relaxation, a space to breathe. It is a space for creativity and connection, for laughter and tears, tea and nourishment on every level. It is a space for mothers and daughters, sisters and neighbours and the friends we are yet to meet. It is a space where you can be however you want to be, where you can play at removing the masks, where you don't say 'I'm fine', you say how you really are, knowing you will be met with love and acceptance.

Claire

A Red Tent is a place where women gather to rest, renew, and often share deep and powerful stories about their lives. The Red Tent is many things to many people. It is a womb-like red fabric space, it is a place where women gather, it is an icon and it is a state of mind.

Isadora Leidenfrost, PhD and ALisa Starkweather [1]

1   Leidenfrost, Isadora, PhD and Starkweather, ALisa.
The Red Tent Movement: A Historical Perspective

Each Red Tent is a unique reflection of the community of women who create it. But these varied spaces all share something in common:

★ the longing for connection and belonging;

★ the sharing of how we are feeling and who we are in our lives at this time;

★ the nourishment of ourselves and each other;

★ the slowing down, changing the pace for rest and replenishment;

★ the simple act of sharing time and space with a group of women;

★ the opportunity to let go of the other responsibilities in our lives;

When women come together, magic happens. We know this to be true from our own experience and in this book we weave together the voices and experiences of many, many women, to create a shared story about the role Red Tents can play in our lives. We have also seen that when these Red Tent communities grow, they can become a beacon to others. This is our hope, our vision, our dream – Red Tents as liberatory community spaces for women around the world.

WELCOME

I had a Red Tent shaped hole in me and I didn't even know it...it felt like coming home.
Zoe

Welcome, we are so glad that you are here with us.

Thank you for showing up wherever you are today in your journey with Red Tents, whether you run a Red Tent already, are just thinking about starting one or are reading this out of curiosity without any intention of running or participating in one. We want you to know that you are welcome and that we invite you to think about Red Tents as a place of welcome that can, with attention and commitment, be intentionally inclusive and accessible to your community.

We invite you to share our vision and travel with us, taking what is useful for you and letting go of the rest. Each Red Tent starts with women sitting in a circle, speaking their name and sharing a short introduction as to where they are right now and how they are. And so that is also how we would like to open this book.

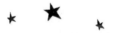

Hi, I'm Mary Ann. The first Red Tent I went to was a gathering of many women, some I already knew well, others I didn't. When I arrived I was invited into a simple circle of women sitting in the small wooden building with a candle in the middle. There were a few red things in the room to indicate a space prepared for us and a simple quiet warm place to be together, to be ourselves, to connect.

I was welcomed. I felt shy and nervous but strangely, not quite so alone as I normally might have, at that time, in a group of women. We'd each brought food to share and there were warm drinks to welcome us. There was something in the space that calmed me and kept me from running away. And as women shared of themselves and of what had brought them there, I began to see myself reflected back, my story echoed. Later in the day during that Red Tent, I slept and found myself able to truly rest in a way I hadn't been able to in months.

It was 2009 and I was at a time in my life when it felt like everything was falling apart. Red Tent spaces held me during that time and punctuated my month like a great big out-breath where I could relax and let go of the multiple challenges I was holding. Being able to share at least some of what I was going through with a group of women helped not just sustain and support me, but also, eventually, to see my way through to making changes.

Seeing and hearing myself in other women's experiences helped me to know on a cellular level that is hard to explain: that although my circumstance were particular to me, the patterns and narratives woven through them were also in some way shared. I was not alone. I had sisters who had had these experiences, had walked these paths, known this grief, this anger, this wrestling, or at least had known something like it. We were kin.

And so it was in the deepest moments of despair in my life that I finally found myself reaching for communities of women, that I too found myself coming home.

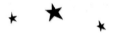

I am Aisha. I always get a tingle when I sit down in a Red Tent and think about a woman doing the very same in another place, feeling connected through this act. This simple way of making time for myself, sharing and enjoying time with other women.

As a child and a teenager, I witnessed how women were objectified, vilified and disregarded. I saw it in my own family, on television and in the ways men treated me. I felt on some level that being a woman was dangerous, weak and full of risk without reward.

Over the years I began to examine this position with a softer gaze. I started making more female friends. I wanted to hear the rich array of stories that made up other people's lives, and to allow wider appreciation to ignite my hope for a celebrated image of women in the future.

Even with some wonderful female friends in my life, the first time I went to a Red Tent I was full to the brim with fear, my heart beating louder than my thoughts. I felt like an imposter rocking on a precipice of something exciting. I knew this feeling well, as I often purposely move towards things that scare me, leaning in to the combined forces of curiosity and terror. I wanted to spend time with other women, although the whole idea of me fully embracing myself as a woman and being vulnerable with them made me recoil.

After my first Red Tent I 'got it'. I had found something more real than the fear and doubt. I had found some sense of connection and acceptance both within myself and with others. I felt passionate about sharing it. I felt the welcome of women to be themselves was something that was missing in society and therefore in countless other women's lives. A year later, I found some women who lived near me who were up for starting a Red Tent. It grew and flourished and took on a life of its own.

1.

A BRIEF HERSTORY
OF RED TENTS

The Red Tent Novel

When we first heard about Red Tents we discovered a loose, diverse and largely uncoordinated movement of women meeting in similar ways. Many we connected to were drawing inspiration from the best-selling novel *The Red Tent* by Anita Diamant, which was first published in 1997. The story spread to a wider audience, in 2014 when a TV mini-series was made based on the book.

The Red Tent is a fictional retelling of a biblical story set in Old Testament times, in which Diamant paints a picture of a Red Tent where women gather, connect and support one another during their menstruation, pregnancy and childbirth. The evocative portrayal of intergenerational sisterhood spoke of being guided and supported through life as part of a community and marking rites of passage through celebration and ritual.

As Isadora Leidenfrost, PhD and ALisa Starkweather say in their book *The Red Tent Movement: A Historical Perspective*, "For many, the story resonated deeply and caused us to question if there (could be) ... a place like this in our society."

Though Anita Diamant wrote a work of fiction, the ideas she included in it drew from what she knew of and had read about women's menstrual rituals and gatherings in Indigenous cultures around the world. In the Lakota Native American tradition, for example, there are moon lodges, which are a creative place where women go for respite when they are bleeding and where elder women give teachings. [1] These are a vital part of the Red Tent lineage.

Whilst Diamant's book has given its name to today's women's spaces and inspired many women, it is not in itself the origin of these ideas but rather a particular format through which they have been communicated. It seems to speak about a shared but hidden longing: for women's space, for ritual, for community. All of which are sorely lacking in many contemporary cultures where patriarchy and whiteness are valued.

These types of traditions held by women to support one another have been deliberately devalued and largely erased. We remember them in large part because many Black and Indigenous women have continued to remember and practice them and have held sacred traditions that affirm women's culture and relationship to one another. There is a long history especially in white and colonised cultures of seeking to wipe out Indigenous and women's rituals and traditions as a means of exerting power and control. For example, prior to the American Indian Religious Freedom Act of 1978, many Native American traditions, customs and rituals were prohibited by law in the US. And in the United Kingdom, where we write from, people thought to be witches, mainly poor or elderly women, accused of practicing magic were violently executed well into the 18th century. [2]

And so in some ways Red Tents are, as ALisa Starkweather and Isadora Leidenfrost, PhD call them, 'reclamation work' [3] helping us connect to lineages and traditions that our cultures have lost, to the practices of our ancestors.

As Madeleine Castro points out, there are also in Red Tents "echoes of consciousness-raising groups that emerged […] during second wave feminism" [4] and we like to think of these groups and the women who created them as part of the lineage of Red Tents also. Like Red Tents, these were groups in which women could sit together, share their struggles and challenges and learn from one another.

---

1   You can hear Beverley Little Thunder speaking with Isadora Leidenfrost, PhD about this as part of her video project here: youtube.com/watch?v=LWyAhSks1GQ

2   One place to read about this is on this website: parliament.uk/about/living-heritage/transformingsociety/private-lives/religion/overview/witchcraft

3   Leidenfrost, Isadora, PhD and Starkweather, ALisa.
The Red Tent Movement: A Historical Perspective

4   Castro, Madeleine. *Introducing the Red Tent: A discursive and critically hopeful exploration of women's circles in a neoliberal postfeminist context.* Sociological Research Online. ISSN 1360-7804

Each stage of feminism has created more space, has pushed out the walls and raised the ceiling for future generations. Part of this process has always been personal as well as political, and personal does not mean just that which applies to us as individuals but also finding ways to meet and support one another on a personal level and to build different practices together. For us Red Tents build on this tradition and are a feminist practice.

And so, in Red Tents we invite you to hold a balance between culture building and culture remembering. These are not binaries. But we can choose to honour lineage and root more solidly into the remnants and surviving pieces of ritual and community in our own cultural and political heritage and we hope that's what you will feel inspired to do through your reading of this book.

Menstrual Retreat

For us, Red Tents are not spaces reserved solely for those who menstruate. However, the idea of a menstrual retreat or refuge is part of the lineage of the Red Tent and so we want to explore it briefly here.

In many cultures, including our own, taboos have developed around menstruation. In some parts of the world this has led to segregation and neglect. In our own, we are still fighting for an acceptance of menstruation and the conversation about it.

In their book, Isadora Leidenfrost, PhD and ALisa Starkweather chart the history of menstrual gatherings as both a blessing and a source of nourishment, as is depicted in the novel, and also as a curse and a means of ostracisation. It is important to note that not all traditions associated with menstruation and other life traditions are empowering and supportive for women.

However, we know that there have been places and times in human history where women's cycles and fertility have been more positively honoured and embraced. There are many communities of women who have remembered this and have traditions of honouring their bleeding time.

Maisie Hill puts it well in her book *Period Power* when she says, "At best a menstrual retreat can provide respite from chores and responsibilities and create time to share in female company, but at worst they are detrimental towards physical and mental health and can risk death. Let's be clear in distinguishing that removing oneself from daily activities to enjoy female company is inherently different from enforced segregation and neglect that is violent and oppressive and based on the belief that women are impure or dangerous."[5]

Camilla Power,[6] an evolutionary anthropologist who looks at early human societies in her work, believes that ancient menstrual rituals may have been part of what enabled them to evolve. She thinks that monthly rituals celebrating bleeding existed in early human groups alongside the lack of overt physical symbols of either ovulation or menstruation, and that this made it difficult to determine when an individual woman was actually bleeding.

Communal rituals that took place when it was a full moon and the skies were bright didn't indicate that female cycles are all aligned and predictable but instead honoured the power of menstruation in general, celebrating it as a rite while keeping the precise timing of menstruation in each individual woman a secret. This served to limit the success of the 'alpha males' who triumphed in our close relatives, gorillas, who procreated and then disappeared. Instead in humans, it was those males who were willing to stick around, who successfully procreated and prospered. And it was they who she believes helped feed their young and thereby supported the necessary brain development in humans as we evolved.

Menstrual rituals may therefore in fact be the oldest tradition with which Red Tents share something in common: they celebrated the female-of-centre experience without needing it to be uniform and were a foundational building block of communal human life.

---

5   Hill, Maisie. *Period Power: Harness Your Hormones and Get Your Cycle Working for You*

6   You can find out more by watching this video: Power, Camilla. "Did Gender Egalitarianism Make Us Human? Or, If Graeber And Wengrow Won't Talk About Sex…" youtube.com/watch?v=xr_7qbI0Gbk

The Red Tent Temple Movement

We first heard about Red Tents from ALisa Starkweather, who is our inspiration in this work. This book would not be here without ALisa and the wisdom and stories she shared with us and many others that have helped seed this movement. ALisa's vision for the Red Tent Temple Movement came to the UK through Women in Power (WIP),[7] a transformational women's initiation programme of which she is a founder. A group of women in the UK, including Nicola Kurk, who is also a WIP founder and inspirational sister of ours, committed in 2009 to holding a Red Tent each month, taking forward ALisa's vision in England. Mary Ann was involved in that commitment, and during that year some new longer-term Red Tents were born.

ALisa's vision was of there being a Red Tent in every village and town. She calls these spaces Red Tent Temples. Like other women who have contributed to an increase in Red Tents, such as DeAnna L'am who advocates for a Red Tent in every neighbourhood, ALisa saw how they could become part of the fabric of our communities. We use the term Red Tents rather than Temples but, like her, we think of them as "a place for us where we can meet each other and at the very same time take care of ourselves and one another."[8] This was – and continues to be – our starting point: that Red Tents are an accessible, community-based initiative for women, supporting them to connect with and take better care of one another.

Another important aspect of the vision that ALisa shared with us was that Red Tents were about *being* rather than *doing*: a place to slow down, to honour the cycles of our lives, connect with the wisdom of other women and share our journeys. These central ideas remain important to us and our vision for Red Tents to this day.

From ALisa we learnt to see that in the simple practice of creating time to listen to one another, journal, share our healing skills and creativity, we were inviting a culture of supportive sharing and connecting amongst women that our cultures so often devalue and disrespect. She also invited us to think about these spaces not just as supportive, fun and replenishing but also as something we desperately needed and which had a role in shifting culture.

---

7   Find out more about Women In Power in the UK at womeninpoweruk.com

8   Find out more about ALisa's work with Red Tents at redtenttemplemovement.com

By creating these spaces and honouring our deep connection we were offering and practicing an alternative to critique and competition between women. We were practicing a way to be in connection and collective care for ourselves and each other. Part and parcel of this was the invitation to stop and be, to breathe, to be in the body and to let go of the busyness and constant doing: to feel and sense, rather than know and judge.

Reflections from ALisa Starkweather

Before reading the Red Tent novel I was influenced by another book, *Circle of Stones: Woman's Journey to Herself* by Judith Duerk in which she poses many questions in the form of "How would your life be different if…?" Each question in the book brings to form a possibility, a place, an experience that could redefine our culture if we brought this to life, if we were held, heard, seen and witnessed in our life experiences.

Anita Diamant's novel, *The Red Tent,* carried many of us deeper than her mere imagination. We remembered home and sisterhood. Her words evoked a bone memory of a place and a time where women were mentored by other women, where the children were cared for, where we gathered with the rhythms of the earth and moon, where we honoured rites of passage in our bleeding, our birthing, our dying, where songs and stories were passed on and images of women as sacred were taught and tended to as part of the culture.

For those whose culture preserved menstrual practices or had years of experience with women as powerful allies, this story was an affirmation rather than a revelation. But for those of us whose lives were being lived out in separation, aloneness, bereft of eldering or any semblance of honouring our bodies, this memory called attention to what had been missing and to what, in many cases, had been completely forgotten.

A longing for home is at its root, nostalgia. We search even without knowing what it means to be held, cared for, to be nourished or tended to. Could it be this place reminds us of sanctuary, a place to grow our children and ourselves within a place of homecoming? For many, the Red Tent is a homecoming.

Starting the Red Tent Directory

While she was part of co-creating a Red Tent in Brighton, Aisha began to have a vision of Red Tents that were grassroots, self-sustaining and visible. She wanted women to feel that they were welcome to start their own and that they could participate in one in their own area.

In part this came out of the experience of Brighton Red Tent, which she co-founded, growing so quickly, with many people travelling to attend it. She felt strongly that the next step from here was to encourage women who came from a distance to come and learn if they wanted to, but to then go back to the place where they lived and start their own, to seed more Red Tents rather than to grow the Brighton Tent larger. This led her to think about how people could be resourced and empowered to start Red Tents themselves and ask what tools they might need to help them do that.

When Aisha looked around, she couldn't find much readily available information about Red Tents. So she began to envisage a visible portal that placed them in the heart of society, made them accessible, tangible and available. With her experience of coordinating a website of ethical business listings, the idea of a directory – that could be an easy hub for Red Tents – began to form. She called out for women who wanted to help support this vision and found Mary Ann who was equally inspired by the idea of making Red Tents more accessible through an online platform and willing to use her nascent web-building skills to help start it. From that moment we set off on this path together.

That vision became a website called the Red Tent Directory that provides a free listing service for Red Tents. Its purpose is to help foster belonging. It's about finding a family of women wherever you lived. It's about finding a sister and being a sister, even if our own family ties are sometimes fragmented. When you know the pain of isolation, it feels as if you never want anyone else to feel it. If there was a way to bridge the divide, then we wanted to find it.

The Directory is our way of helping share what women were already doing. We also wanted to make the idea of Red Tents more accessible and to simplify it, so any woman could create or join a Tent. To us, this was a co-created grassroots movement from the very start, and we wanted to help facilitate that.

Red Tents are a loose global movement of community and connection and we were only one voice within it. We saw our role as nourishing and supporting women to create gatherings, so we actively chose not to control or restrict what was happening or to have any way of vetting or authenticating the Tents that wanted to list with us. To this end, we deliberately only had a few policies about the nature of the Red Tents we listed.

When we launched the site in December 2012, we listed just four Tents. In fact, in the beginning we actually had to beg people to list with us, to believe in our idea of a listing site at all! We knew there were a number of Red Tents running but we found that knowledge was spreading largely by word of mouth and that there was some reluctance initially about being more visible. Some questioned why an online presence made sense for such personal gatherings but we felt committed to making visible what was happening so that more women could be invited into Red Tents.

We had initially envisaged the Directory as a UK listing site, but we soon had a request from our WIP sisters in France and so we listed their Tent in Paris too. As our commitment to this work grew and developed, we became aware of many other Red Tents beyond those inspired by ALisa. The Tents we listed soon expanded to Spain, Portugal and Germany and eventually in 2013 we began to list any Red Tent within Europe. Recently we became a worldwide listing site and invite Tents from anywhere in the world to list on our Directory. At the time of writing, there are over two hundred Red Tents all around the world listed with us!

As a result of the many, many women who began to contact us, we became increasingly aware that Red Tents take many forms. We welcomed those who had been inspired in other ways and didn't necessarily know of ALisa, to list their Red Tents on the site we had created. The Red Tent Directory, therefore, lists Red Tents which have varied stories about how and why they started and who and what they have been inspired by.

As time went by, we also realised that we needed to define exactly what Red Tents were so we could make decisions about listings and as a result of much discussion between us and with women who list on our site, we came to agree that we would list Red Tents that fulfil the following criteria:

★ women meeting and holding a circle where each woman gets time and space to speak without discussion or debate;

★ women meeting regularly at an agreed time and place;

★ gatherings which are either free or donation-based to cover room hire or tea with the amount ideally left to the discretion of the donor;

★ circles which respond to the wishes of those present rather than primarily running workshops, trainings or any deliberate kind of personal development.

Red Tents are a place to be seen and heard as women and enjoy life. It's a place of support and encouragement, where you can recharge and enjoy the company of other women. A place you can feel safe and appreciated in a non-judgemental, caring space. A place to explore interests and new possibilities, learn from each other and feel uplifted.
Julia

As our vision took root, we also began to offer guidance and mentoring to help support conversations to take place within Red Tents so they could adapt and emerge as communities shifted and grew.

Over the years we have worked with over twenty volunteers and supported dozens of women on the phone and by email to establish, run and also, in some cases, close Red Tents. We have provided support with everything from envisioning and holding, to promotion and conflict resolution, and we have learnt a lot along the way about the things that seem to make Red Tents flourish and grow. This book is our attempt to share our learning from that journey and to articulate our vision for Red Tents.

Articulating a vision wasn't something we set out to do at the beginning of the project – we just planned to provide a listing service which would make Red Tents visible and help this growing practice be *seen*. But, over time, we have felt more and more called to share the vision that has emerged from our experience of being in touch with so many Red Tents. It is not so much *our* vision, but a vision emerging from the loosely coordinated movement we reflect on the Directory website, a vision of women gathering across different countries within their communities to create a web of connection and support.

2.

AN EMERGING VISION

Red Tent to me is creating a safe space where women can come as they are and just 'be'. Where they can be open and honest and feel that shared experience with other women without judgement.

Leigh-Anne

We think of Red Tents as community-held spaces where women can come to connect with each other in ways that aren't necessarily common or familiar to us. And we think of the practice of doing this, of meeting each other monthly to share, and rest, as something that allows us to connect to one another in a different kind of way from what we might be used to. Connecting by intentionally listening and deliberately seeking not to 'fix' or critique. Doing this we think can be a liberatory practice that helps support change in our lives and in our world.

Fundamentally this book is a celebration of this movement and the power we think it has to support and transform. And it is also meant as an invitation, if you haven't yet, to join in! In this book, as well as inspiration and practical learning, we have included some questions and practices to support you, as well as discussion about some of the challenges we know Red Tents face.

A few years ago, we developed and launched a free toolkit that we made available on our website in which we began to share our learning about things women were finding effective in creating Red Tents. The toolkit has since been downloaded over 1400 times.

In this book we go beyond that toolkit and lay out our vision for collective leadership of Red Tents and for challenging harm and injustice in this diverse and multi-faceted movement. We do so in the spirit not of making it something we take any particular leadership of, but of articulating what we think and believe is possible. We hope in doing so we will offer support and guidance to help others develop Red Tents and contribute to what is truly an organic, fluid and dynamic collective movement in a way that enables Red Tents to become spaces in which we develop liberatory practices of collective care.

Leading together (as we suggest you do) resists the cult of the individual so prominent in so-called western culture at this point in time and the ways in which patriarchy tends to divide all those oppressed by gender binaries. We want to invite you to think about liberating ourselves by doing this together. We know this is often hard because we are so conditioned to go it alone and to build walls between ourselves. But as we hope you will learn through the pages of this book, doing things together and embracing our differences can be truly rewarding.

Social Justice and Inclusion by Design

From the very start of our journey together with this work, we have been in conversation about what inclusion means and could look like in Red Tent spaces, though we by no means have all of the answers.

We want to start by acknowledging that we write as two white, relatively privileged women living in the United Kingdom, a country that has a significant history of colonialism and exploitation. And we write with an awareness that many of the practices and traditions which Red Tents draw upon or remember are those that originate in or have been maintained by Indigenous communities and communities of colour. We believe that colonial white supremacy and patriarchy have suppressed and distorted many ways women have had of meeting and supporting one another. As a result, many of us have lost these traditions and have little living memory of ways of honouring life stages and transitions. Meanwhile many Black and Indigenous people of colour have held onto and nurtured these traditions. Through the pages of this book we will be inviting you to honour those lineages and legacies, to name where you have learnt the practices from you use in Red Tent spaces, the communities that have made it possible for us to remember them and also to support them financially where possible.

As Resmaa Menakem says, white people who commit to anti-racism "must build culture, because culture trumps almost everything else" [1] and so, as two white women balancing our desire to share these ideas and an awareness of our own privilege, we invite you to think of Red Tents as a collective culture-building practice.

We know that if we don't name the structural inequities showing up in Red Tents they can easily become examples of an exclusive kind of space dominated by what Layla Saad has called "spiritual white women" – women who engage in spirituality without acknowledging the Indigenous roots of the spirituality we engage with or the inequities in the world and the ways in which they show up in spiritual and collective practice.

As she says, what can happen is that we "believe that the best thing they [we] can do is just focus on being a good and loving person, and serving their [our largely white] audience and sending love and light instead of actually speaking up". [2]

We are very clear that we don't want any part in perpetuating Red Tents that ignore the inequities in the world and the lineages we draw from. And so our own love for the Red Tent as a form for women to connect and be with one another, is coupled with a commitment to make this book a call to women who run or would like to run Red Tents to see their Red Tents as a part of a practice of collective healing and liberation. To make holding Red Tents a practice in which we support one another to transform how we relate to each other and commit to speaking up about injustice.

This means wrestling with all the forms of oppression present in our lives that will show up in Red Tents, and it means building our awareness so that we can make our practice of running and holding Red Tents more liberatory. Actively seeking to challenge the harm and injustice that can show up in Red Tent spaces is one small way of being in the practice of resisting oppressive systems in our ways of being together. We discover the joy of a practice that challenges racism, transphobia, homophobia, classism, fatphobia, ageism and ableism and the benefits that this can bring us as a collective. We can do this in the rituals and spaces we create, speaking through our actions as well as our words.

It is our belief that if your Red Tent isn't on a pathway to seek to heal injustice, you are likely inadvertently perpetuating it. And so, we want to

---

1   Menakem, Resmaa. *My Grandmother's Hands: Racialized Trauma and the Pathway to Mending our Hearts and Bodies*

2   You can read Layla Saad's article about this on her website: laylafsaad.com/poetry-prose/white-women-white-supremacy-1

invite you, whether or not you have done so in the past, to consider how to make your Red Tent a place where you intentionally seek not to replicate oppressive systems and instead establish a collective practice of care that can help create change.

When we say *women* on our website and in this work, we were initially thinking of women who identify as women and use the pronouns she/her. However, we have continued to be challenged to think more about gender as a construct and have come to believe that Red Tents should be spaces for cisgender women, transgender women, non-binary trans femme, intersex and non-binary people.

Therefore, we are writing from a feminist perspective about gatherings orientated towards those who are female-of-centre, and who self-identify as women or queer, rather than writing specifically for those who were assigned the gender 'woman' at birth or who bleed. And so, while the Red Tent is related in some ways to traditions of menstrual rituals, as we document in more detail in the next chapter, Red Tent gatherings are not in our view specifically for those who bleed. Those who no longer bleed or have never menstruated should, we think, be welcomed to them.

Gender is a complex cultural, as well as biological, construct. Tents can be inclusive spaces which are richer for providing space for the full spectrum of lived experiences. In this book we invite you to commit to the inclusion of trans and non-binary people in any Red Tents that you attend or run and to consider how you replicate or resist the gender binary. In the words of Julia Serano, "There are countless experiences that can shape a woman's gendered experiences: being socialized as a girl (or not), experiencing menstruation and menopause (or not), becoming pregnant and giving birth (or not), becoming a mother (or not), having a career outside of the home (or not), having a husband (or a wife or neither), and so on. Women's lives are also greatly shaped by additional factors such as race, age, ability, sexual orientation, economic class, and so on. While each of these individual experiences are shared by many women – and each is rightfully considered a 'women's issue' – it would be foolish for anyone to claim that any one of these was a prerequisite for calling oneself a woman. So long as we refuse to accept that 'woman' is a holistic concept, one that includes all people who experience themselves as women, our concept of womanhood will remain a mere re-flection of our own personal experiences and biases rather than something based in the truly diverse world that surrounds us."[3]

For the purposes of this book, we will use the language of *woman* and *women* in place of listing all gender identities for ease and flow. However where we want you to consider many voices within the context of the specific and often intersectional marginalisation we all experience at this point in human history we will specify gender terms and identities for clarity. We also know that, within this, some specific groups of women may choose to gather in a dedicated space and so Red Tents that are, for example, specifically for women of colour, older women, girls and so on, are also ideas we will explore in the pages of this book. We think of dedicated spaces like this as important pieces of a bigger puzzle. Throughout the book we will share REFLECTIVE QUESTIONS to deepen your own enquiry. These can be used for discussion with a sister or Red Tent holding group, or simply for your own reflection.

Table of Terms

Language we have chosen to use to describe racialised groups in this book is intended to recognise that no term is perfect and, in using these terms, we are seeking to describe the reality of an unjust and unacceptable system of organising human life. There are many other terms in use and many other ways in which we could have done this. We don't mean to infer that these are the only ways to describe racialised groups, indeed we acknowledge that within terms like 'people of colour' there is a huge range of human diversity that, if we are not careful, can be erased by blanket terms like these. Therefore, consider using more detailed ways of describing individual people and their heritage when and if you can.

* BIPOC – Black, Indigenous and people of colour.

* Black – people of colour of African heritage (may also be mixed). This term is capitalised throughout the book deliberately to acknowledge Blackness as a specific identity.

* Brown – people of colour who do not identify as Black.

---

3   Serano, Julia. *Whipping Girl: A Transsexual Woman on Sexism and the Scapegoating of Femininity*

* Mixed – someone of dual heritage.

* Native – Indigenous people, especially on Turtle Island (so-called US and Canada).

* POC/WOC – people of colour/women of colour.

* White – someone raced as white – may include those of mixed heritage who 'look white', sometimes called 'white-passing'.

When discussing gender, we want to name the multiple expressions within the gender spectrum. However, we envisage that in time there will be additional terms and identities that are not included in this book or listed here.

* AFAB – people assigned female at birth.

* Cisgender/cis – people whose gender identity matches their sex assigned at birth.

* Femme – people who identify with aspects coded as feminine while not necessarily a female gender.

* Female-of-Centre – a word that indicates a range of terms of gender identity and gender presentation for people who present, understand themselves, and/or relate to others in a more feminine way, but don't necessarily identify as women.

* Genderqueer/gender-nonconforming/gender diverse – people who are intersex or non-binary and identify outside of the gender binary.

* Intersex – people whose anatomy, chromosomes or physiology differ from contemporary cultural stereotypes of what constitute expected patterns of male and female.

* Non-binary – people who choose to not identify with a gender relating to a binary spectrum.

* Queer – people of sexual and gender-nonconforming identities. Also used to describe gender diverse and norm-challenging ideas.

* Transgender/trans – people whose gender identity does not match their sex assigned at birth.

Radical Work

For me, the Red Tent is a radical space. 'Radical' coming from 'root' – it is a grassroots movement, providing a place for female identifying people to feel a sense of belonging, a sense of home. It is in acknowledging that Red Tents aren't always experienced in this way for everyone that I realise the work I (and those of us who are part of the Red Tent movement) still have to do to live up to this vision.

How can we create a place where we can question the structures that hold us, and allow the female voice to be truly heard, to feel valued, to feel safe?

In the Red Tent we can explore ideas that may have been dismissed or silenced. By engaging with and celebrating these ideas, we give them weight and strength, knowing that they have been celebrated before.

The Red Tent is a place where I can let go of my roles, my sense of obligation and what is expected of me and simply be.

The Red Tent is a place to connect with women from the past, present and future, where we can feel our interwoven threads and celebrate allyship.

*The fact that the Red Tent is a co-creative space, that no money is involved, that it is a space for acceptance and tolerance, that it provides a place where we can feel a true sense of sisterhood and what it is to **be** together... All of these things, for me, define the Red Tent gatherings as a radical act in the face of the capitalist, patriarchal constructs that dominate western culture.*

Lily

When we set out to create the spaces that our culture has not necessarily gifted us, the path is rewarding but not always easy. We want you to know and remember that creating spaces for women to share their journeys with each other is radical work that challenges the status quo in cultures that often marginalise women's stories and experiences. In fact, by being part of this movement, even by simply picking up and reading this book, you are part of something which, in small and everyday ways, is about shifting the way in which women relate to one another and show up in their lives.

Red Tents, by design, move us away from the kind of connections women have, where we feel in competition or where we feel we need to prove ourselves. Red Tents are spaces where we deliberately invite permission to just *be* and intentionally cultivate a culture between women of connection, cooperation and mutual support and solidarity. The Red Tent is where we can let go and be heard and hear one another.

A sense of collective sisterhood can be cultivated in these spaces, whatever our roles and responsibilities in the rest of our lives.

We envision Red Tents as being:

* held collectively, either by a small group or by a woman who is held within a wider community, with a structure that intentionally invites connection, cooperation, mutual support and solidarity, as opposed to competition;

* community spaces, co-created by women who share community in some way, whether geographically or in a particular setting;

* spaces of collective care, healing and welcome that practice acknowledging harm and shifting culture, seeking not to perpetuate injustice.

We are aware that Red Tents come in many shapes, sizes and forms. Not all are held communally, their structures and practices vary. Many are led by passionate women who take individual responsibility for creating and holding them.

Our vision is not intended to critique any other practice that is out there. We welcome all of what is. And, at the same time, we want to invite you to think about the possibility of Red Tents that are held collectively, that allow each and every member to rest and connect, that don't rely so much on the leadership of an individual woman, but that instead lean in to what women might create together.

This possibility and practice of creating Red Tents together, which gives us a collective space to lean in to, to connect with one another and to build our muscle for connection, support and solidarity, is what the rest of this book is about.

Creating Red Tents like this isn't always easy, because the simple act of doing so challenges what we have learned about being and working together. It means letting go of our agendas and our assumptions. It means dealing with challenges and conflicts when they arise, and committing to the value of a collective approach, of inviting a new paradigm of what is possible.

We know it is possible and through the pages of this book we will share stories from different Red Tents to give you a window on these possibilities and ideas to get started with and jump off from in your own Red Tent community.

Menstruation Does Not Define Womanhood

I wonder if the dominant depiction of the Red Tent as connected to women's bodies – menstruation, wombs, etc. – might be somewhat alienating to differing types of women such as trans women and non-binary individuals? This also potentially connects to a unified idea of womanhood. Whilst there are experiences that women (of all differing kinds) might share, women are not one homogenous lump, and there are real, lived intersectional differences such as race, ethnicity, age, sexuality, (dis)ability, class but also embodiment. These affect women in different ways and circles have the potential to be able to allow for, hear and even value these differences. But are circles attracting and welcoming diverse types of women and non-binary individuals?

None of this is to deny the need for spaces to discuss the realities of women's bodies. In contexts where women's bodies have been scrutinised, controlled, sexualised, violated and subjugated by patriarchal systems in all kinds of ways, I think it is important that there is a context in which sexuality and women's bodies are reclaimed, including spaces where menstruation can be normalised. However, I don't think that this should be at the expense of differing experiences of womanhood, which would include diverse experiences of embodiment too. The idea of a 'symbolic womb space' can be useful here in that it recognises a 'feminine energy' without prescribing what this is exactly.

Madeleine

The Red Tent is about welcoming and accepting women for who they are and how they are in that moment. It is about supporting and allowing women to be all of who they are, both multi-layered and holding paradoxes. Menstruating may be one part of the experience of womanhood, but not the whole picture. Framing menstruation as the only narrative that unites women together oversimplifies and limits our lived experiences.

Almost all the Tents we know of welcome women who have stopped bleeding because they have passed through menopause or those who have never cycled at all. There are also women attending Tents who are not currently cycling due to pregnancy, birth or because they are taking the contraceptive pill. Many Tents have also created specific spaces for women at specific points in their lives including, Tents for girls or for women who have passed through the menopause. There is more about these later in the book.

That said, if you are a cisgender woman menstruation may well be hugely important to you in terms of your insight into yourself and your identity and tracking your cycle may well provide many eureka moments. [4] For you, having a regular cycle may be one of the key defining aspects of how you experience yourself as a woman.

Learning about the potential lessons within my menstrual cycle as an adult changed my relationship to pain and rest. I had often felt like my body was failing me by hurting and shedding blood each month. More often than not I felt completely dislocated from my physical self and ignored or numbed out sensations of discomfort.

Finding that I could view my periods as a map to navigate the landscape of my month gave me much needed tools. I found a sense of power in observing the fluctuations of mood and a way to harness aspects of these changes to activate parts of my life. For example, the nervous energy I feel pre-period helps me to organise, tidy and declutter in my home, my life and my work. It is very different from the more creative energy I feel early in my period where I can make and build things and have lots of ideas fermenting under the surface.

I found through observing and learning about my cycle that the pain I experienced during the bleeding time provided an opportunity to slow down, a call for self-care. I found that I had an opportunity to not ignore

---

4   There are many resources that can help you learn how to do this including *Moon Time, Reaching for the Moon, Period Power, Wild Power* and *Code Red* all of which are included in the Resources section at the end of this book.

what was happening and push through, but to learn to listen. Now I try to organise my diary with a sense of my cycle and even when I do continue at a pace during my period, I try to remember I need some kindness, however I can bring that in.

Aisha

It is still taboo in many places to tell colleagues or friends that you are not feeling very well due to changes in your body, be that monthly bleeds, endometriosis, menopause or transitioning to another gender. Campaigning for reproductive rights is also dangerous in many parts of the world. In this context many of us learn from a young age that periods are not a subject that can be openly discussed. When menstruation interferes with our education or life plans, we may make other excuses of a headache or stomach upset when we need to go home early or not be in work at all, or find ourselves pushing on through despite an inner knowing that we need to rest.

I started menstruating at 10, earlier than many of the girls around me. I expected it in some ways because my mum, who also 'started early' had explained what would happen and why, but I did feel that no one understood and that I had to hide my bleeding and just get on with things. The other kids teased me for being younger than them and yet I had this great flood of red blood coming out of me. It didn't seem fair.

Mary Ann

As Tessa shares below, it forms a part of her Red Tent to openly mention where you are in your menstrual cycle, thereby creating one place in women's lives that they can voice this in a judgement-free setting. Practicing this for ourselves and amongst ourselves in Red Tents can help us to bring this openness to the rest of our lives.

Women come in alone, or in pairs or threes and find a space. They often like to sit in the same spot each time we gather. They get a hot drink and chat until everyone has arrived. Then we start with introductions – name, day of cycle if they know and if they're cycling, maybe a couple of

27

words on how their day has been.
Tessa

As two cisgender women we do not see our experience of menstruating as being the defining thing that makes us a woman. Rather menstruation is one aspect of our lives which, both being in our 40s now, has been consistent for many years and which we know is a chapter that may soon begin to draw to a close for us. But if having a monthly cycle was the precursor to being accepted as a woman, then anyone who is not menstruating due to illness or medical intervention would no longer be a woman. If a woman is only considered a woman because she knows the sensations and manifestations of menstruating, then women who never have periods for medical reasons could not be considered women, nor hold the pronoun *she* or join women-only spaces.

In writing this book we have spoken to trans women and intersex and non-binary people who have shared feeling excluded and *othered* by the focus on the normative expectations of the female body. We have learnt that clear biological distinctions are only possible if we ignore the diverse experience of people's medical, physical and emotional experiences and needs. And we have come to understand that the focus on menstruation as central to the definition of being a woman often makes trans women feel that they are not and will never be accepted as female. This is hurtful, oppressive and diminishing.

It was very natural and felt rich, right and powerful for us when we explored menstruation and menopause and rites of passage with trans women and girls and non-binary participants present, sharing their own experiences. We reflected on our language so that everyone there would feel that this was a space they felt seen and heard in – I feel this has deepened and enhanced our offering and our understanding and it adds so much to the circles and the learning. Trans women often know lots about hormones and add insight and wisdom and we all learn more…plus the women who are trans in our group often follow the moon cycles and often there are many women in the group who haven't got wombs or don't bleed, so we let everyone speak from their own experience. I remember in one circle gathering a cis woman said to a trans woman "You have taught me so much about being a woman and what it means". This can be the reality of what more inclusive spaces can look and feel like. We don't always get it right but that shouldn't deter us from trying.

Clare

When we spoke to Kim, who identifies as non-binary, they shared their experience of menstruating with us:

From a personal perspective, I've never attached womanhood or feminin-ity to my menses or, indeed, any part of my existence. I knew I wasn't a girl from about the age of three, but it was almost 30 more years before I fully understood what that meant. I was what they would call a "late bloomer". I didn't get my first period until I was 17. It was a struggle navigating this aspect of my life in part due to the shame and stigma attached to periods in general and with being a working-class individual with limited access to sanitary products.

Kim

In this book – and in the practice we are sharing for creating Red Tent spaces – we encourage a conscious act of claiming space for ourselves which models retreat time and sisterly support as an act of cultural resistance to a culture that seems to keep us both busy and disconnected from one another.

What we want to make clear is that in the wider context of being a woman we can look beyond our biological body to be inclusive of everyone, with-out denying anyone's personal experience. Understanding that biology does not define womanhood does not negate our own experience of our bodies and the power we might have found in understanding different facets of them. Or our own unique ways of exploring the impact of hormones or developing a personal understanding of our own menstrual cycles. It simply invites us to broaden our understanding of the different experiences others have and understand that actually, we are not all the same, nor are we ex-periencing our bodies in the same way. Bringing this acknowledgement of difference rather than an assumption of sameness to Red Tent spaces is, we believe, critically important.

REFLECTIVE QUESTIONS

★ What has this section brought up for you about your own relationship to your body?

★ What has it brought up for you about ideas and experiences of womanhood and menstruation?

★ How might you change your practice as a result?

★ What challenges you about it?

★ What can you do to broaden your knowledge of other peoples lived experiences?

What We Are Up Against

To me Red Tents are a place where women can relax and feel their power: their personal power and their collective power. I find it hard to explain what goes on, because it is powerful at many levels. I think it is something to be experienced. We can attempt to put it into words, but the experience is much more than that.

Juliet

In different cultures and communities different things are considered taboo, but most of us grew up learning that there were certain things it was not safe to talk about.

Many women come to the Red Tent used to not speaking of the things that affect them deeply: their life experiences, their bodies, their lives. Women come to the Red Tent unsure how they could ever openly share experiences like failure, frustration or loneliness or to speak about things like rape, miscarriage, sexual violence, FGM and incest that our societies have, in various different ways, taught us to hide. It is not always easy to find the courage to answer the question of "how are you?" or "tell me about your life…" with real honesty.

Red Tents, at their simplest, are about creating spaces to break our silence with each other. To break it in a held and confidential space. This happens, often slowly and over time, because in Red Tents we deliberately give each woman an opportunity to share whatever is present for her on that day, in that moment. An uninterrupted space in which to share whatever she might choose to in the company of other women. And whilst there is no rush to speak the 'unspeakable', sometimes, we have found, it helps more than we ever expected. In fact, in Red Tents we have found, sometimes to our own amazement, that we tell each other stories of the things we would hide. From our desires, to our waist sizes. From our first bleeds to our experiences of violence.

For me, the Red Tent is a place to be heard, to be healed, to feel the release of pent up feelings which cannot be expressed safely anywhere else. I learn from the stories shared and carry their lessons home.

Carla

The silencing of women, which manifests in many ways, including when women are not listened to, are asked to stay quiet, are overlooked for positions and continue to be under-represented in many parts of our societies has been the predominant social model within patriarchy for centuries perhaps millennia.

In the culture in which we both live, in contemporary Britain, it is clear that this silencing is often exacerbated by inequality. Our culture further silences those identifying as women who are Black, Indigenous and people of colour, and those who do not have access to economic or social privileges such as education and resources. This has, we believe, been part of a strategy to maintain the status quo, a status quo in which power and resources have been largely concentrated in the hands of men and specifically also in the hands of people raced as white.

We want to be clear that when we say this, we don't mean to accuse specific white men of anything. We both identify as white, live with cis white men, and are both mothers to white male children. We love them and honour them and are deeply grateful to our partners for the support they have offered us in this work. But when we say this, we are describing a system that we have all been living with in which white men are assumed to be superior to everyone else and therefore experience more opportunity and comfort. And in which those of us with privilege benefit from the oppression of others, often in ways we don't see. A system in which, for example, Black, Indigenous and people of colour have to try harder than white people do to achieve the same things. And the more intersections of marginalisation that a person has to deal with, the harder their experience gets. We need to talk about the impact of this and explore how we can each be part of creating change.

From my own experience, most Red Tents I attended were run by white women who were British, married, employed, between thirty and forty and living in a good area with a good home set up. How does this represent all of us? I was not average when I set up my Red Tent: I am Black, a foreigner in the UK, employed and living in a one-bedroom flat with my son, divorced and a single parent. I hoped I would attract a similar pool of women and it felt good. But I wanted to create a space that could welcome all the women – the middle class, the less comfortable, the domestic abuse survivor, the one who is in a forced marriage. My point is lack of representation creates no representation at all and that's a big issue, a kind of Catch-22 situation.

Pascale

White supremacy, a powerful idea, in operation around the world, erases other cultural practices in multiple different ways. For us Red Tents are part of how we can build alternative cultural practices that can help us to address these things and in doing so to acknowledge that nothing is really new. We are aware that in many Indigenous cultures, women have held on to traditions that have helped them support one another and themselves in ways that most women in the white British culture we know best largely have not.

And so, in creating Red Tent spaces we may be calling back to traditions our ancestors had but which we, as white women, can no longer remember clearly. Meanwhile, we may deliberately or inadvertently be borrowing from cultures that have preserved women's traditions in ways that constitute cultural appropriation – where we take a practice as our own without acknowledgement or accountability.

This is what we are up against.

Meanwhile, the impact of the ways in which patriarchy silences women means that many women have learnt to keep quiet, to toe the line, to accept things and to have our voices under-represented throughout public life. Moreover, in many places around the world, women are busy and expected to do the lion's share of caring for the old and young, the real work of sustaining our existence. And it is often poorer, more marginalised women who also take on care roles for wealthier women. When we are busy with that to the point of exhaustion, it feeds our silence about all the ways in which the systems we are living in and with are not working for us.

This is what we are up against.

Within the framework of patriarchy, women are invited to stay in the home, to connect less with one another, to compete with rather than support one another. This manifests in many different ways and lives within us when we struggle to connect and instead see each other as a competitor.

Our socialisation has included an invitation to compete over how we look, what we can achieve both at home and at work (how successful we are, how tidy our homes are and so on). To be the best wife, the good girl, the ideal woman, is to care for house, home and family. We are encouraged to be happy with our lot and not make too much noise.

This is what we are up against.

We may have friendships with each other, but they don't always feel very challenging to the status quo. Perhaps you, like us, have had the experience of realising you are not in fact telling your dear friends how you actually feel, that even for them, there is a way in which you are curating how you show up.

Women have been silenced and we have, in our own ways, been formed by this culture and so most of us are, to some extent, complicit in it. We have experienced the devaluation of the feminine in our society where it has become synonymous with inferior. We have colluded with the internalised misogyny of seeing anything related to women as less worthy, less serious or less valuable. [5] We have invalidated our feelings, our intuition and our power.

We have feared writing this book because it feels like resistance. We have feared sharing our voices in case someone shoots us down. We have wondered whether it is really the right thing for us to show up in this way. We have critiqued ourselves again and again.

This is what we are up against.

When it comes to our bodies and to our bleeding, we have been socialised to stay silent about our experiences. Many of us were not brought up to feel empowered about our bodies and the changes they go through.

My first moon came when I was about thirteen. I was young and I was carefree. My mum, I mean she's amazing, but she didn't really prepare me for what periods would be like... So I discovered by myself and I didn't really acknowledge them. I wasn't happy or angry I was just quite indifferent to be honest... I think I started to be more interested in my periods before getting pregnant, and a lot more after. And now in my thirties, I've really started to appreciate them.

It's allowing me to be more connected to my body. I feel when it's coming [whereas] before I didn't even know... My body would feel the same to me 28 days a month, but now it's different. Now I know I'm not the same. I know my body's heavier and more sensitive. I couldn't feel any of this before. I was busy trying to make money, trying to please people, all this [kind of] thing. And that disconnected me from myself. So I feel

5 Serano, Julia. *Whipping Girl: A Transsexual Woman on Sexism and the Scapegoating of Femininity*

something has changed in my body.

I think when we reconnect fully to the body and to what the body does, you know, whatever it does, we feel much stronger, we feel empowered, we feel full, we feel aligned. And then we can help other women to feel the same.

Pascale

Many of us were not encouraged to understand our cycles, to have knowledge of our fertility or lack of, to navigate feeling misgendered or outside of the societal norms of gender. There was so much we didn't know that could have helped us to work with our bodies instead of against them.

I didn't fit, because my body doesn't fit the normalised narratives. They are particularly restrictive because they lead us to believe that there are types and idealised certainties and that then devalues everyone, everyone that doesn't fit that…people like me.

Lu

The period poverty movement is finally helping to explode and explore taboos around menstruation and is able to share that with a wider audience, thanks to social media and the possibilities of global communication. Some of the organisations who are part of this movement are also providing support across the intersections of inequality for cisgender and transgender women, and gender non-conforming people and the lived experiences of differing challenges.[6] We honour the many women who are doing this work, raising their voices and rejecting the things that keep us silent about our own lives or would seem to have power over us.

Liberating ourselves from the biological construct of gender does not mean diminishing our physical lived experiences but instead honouring their diversity, the range of ways to be women, to be female and to challenge a patriarchal status quo.

The history of our oppression is linked to the history of our exploitation. In our culture we see the value of growth at all costs, the constant obsession

6 Including Bloody Good Period bloodygoodperiod.com

with things becoming bigger and better, the unspoken horror of our colonial history and of white supremacy which has colonised land and bodies and taken them for our profit for centuries.

As white women born into a colonising culture, we recognise ourselves as both oppressor and oppressed and in this work we try to stay conscious of that as we navigate this paradox. We have significant privilege and we also experience a sense of having been silenced. We live in a culture and nation that colonised a large part of the world in living memory and has yet to make reparation for that past.

Through this work we seek to encourage you and to encourage ourselves to build ways of relating to one another that challenge assumed and unearned privilege. We invite you to think about how you might make reparation through the honouring of those who have preserved traditions and offer material support to them where that feels possible.

We view gender as a social construct distinct from our biology. Biology has, in so many ways, been used against us. Trans and queer women and people outside of the binary have been excluded from the gendered spaces in our society in a way that is meant to divide rather than to serve and uplift us. The oppressive construct of gender, is part of a wider oppressive and exclusionary mindset, as Alison Phipps expresses so well in *Me, Not You: The Trouble with Mainstream Feminism:* "It is impossible to disentangle the war against 'gender ideology' from the widespread racism and anti-immigrant sentiment directed at other Others also seen as threats. 'Taking our country back' and 'making it great again' means closing our doors against, expelling or assimilating anyone who dares to produce, reproduce or think differently. It means reasserting geographical and ideological borders: defending the normatively gendered, cis, white, enabled and 'economically productive' capitalist body against those on the outside."

The resources of our earth, the very things that sustain and nourish us, have been exploited to such an extent that our very existence is under deep threat. We have been socialised into cultures that implicitly value growth over rest and cyclical rejuvenation. We are participating willingly in our own demise at the altar of profit for the few.

The urge to exploit and control has extended to our bodies, to the shocking extent of sexual and domestic violence on our planet. We are exploited, we exploit ourselves. Our planet is exploited and we feel powerless to stop it.

This is what we are up against.

Stepping into Our Power

We see the Red Tent work we do in the context of a world in need of radical change. As we move through Covid-19 (at the time of writing this book) we are learning the sacredness of our connections to one another and seeing too that building networks of support and care for each other may be all that we have. In other words, this is not just women meeting to talk about 'things like periods', but rather this is a potentially radical structure, a feminist act and a call to the practice of doing things differently.

We believe that in the framework of patriarchy we have been taught that we are not supposed to support each other and that Red Tents are an everyday radical practice of women rejecting and disrupting this bullshit. Red Tents can be a small but important part of the solution – the movement against this.

We situate our work within a framework of power in which power is not just the power that has been used to exploit or suppress us but the power we have together and within ourselves.[7] Through the connections we build in Red Tents we seek to orient ourselves towards a kind of power with and within that can help us to be a humble and small part of the solutions to these complex and often seemingly overwhelming global problems.

We have seen women experience the impact of these problems on their bodies and seen it manifest as depression, exhaustion, self-harm and illness. We have felt ourselves internalise misogyny and patriarchy and act against other women and against our own interests. But we also believe that we can use our power positively to be a force for change.

The Red Tent Movement is a call to revolutionary friendship with one another, to the radical act of carving space for ourselves in the company of each other. And to a commitment to that which is system-challenging by our practice.

The Red Tent is a place to drop down our defences and be truly seen by the women in our community. It is an opportunity to practice fiercely and courageously speaking our truth from our deepest vulnerability and to be welcomed with open arms when we do. It is our chance to create the world

7   Lisa VeneKlasen, "Last Word – How does Change Happen?" (2006), justassociates.org/sites/justassociates.org/files/development_journal.veneklasen_0.pdf

we long for together.
Mandy

We are all operating under capitalist white supremacist patriarchy right now and in cultures that are racist, transphobic, and ableist. We have seen how the culture we are living in can challenge us in this work.

How it trips us up.

How we can feel compelled to lead individually rather than to build together.

How we can find ourselves creating spaces that only feel safe to white women.

How we can find that questions of money and resources plague us and challenge our collective structures.

How we make assumptions that diversity is catered for without ever asking how others feel.

How we close off from conflict or questions or accountability.

How we internalise all the ways we have been critiqued.

Perhaps patriarchy, capitalism and white supremacy are in their early dying days. Perhaps we are seeds of a new tomorrow in this work. But that is by no means a certainty in these precarious moments: change takes, and will take, time. For now, we have to operate in these systems at least to some extent in order to continue to meet this moment. And so, questions of resourcing are real. Questions of how we can work together are meaningful. Questions of structure and leadership become key.

How do we imagine the structures that can hold us when what we are seeking is radically different from what we know?

We are imagining something different and it takes a commitment to trial and error, a willingness to get it wrong sometimes and to stop something and start afresh.

This book is a guide for you in your own discovery…but it's not a *step by step, this is simple if you follow the instructions to the letter* kind of guide. Instead, it's full of reflections and questions offered to support your own exploration, accompanied by the stories and reflections of many women in our communities who have walked this Red Tent path too. Consider it a community between paper covers. Seeds of possibility that need your presence, your awareness, your lived-out actions to grow.

REFLECTIVE QUESTIONS

★ How have you experienced being silenced in your life?

★ What do you no longer want to be silent about?

★ How might Red Tent friendships support you to be revolutionary?

★ What oppressions do you experience and how have you internalised them?

★ Where do you notice privilege in yourself and your life?

★ What, if anything, is challenging to you about thinking about all of this?

PART TWO

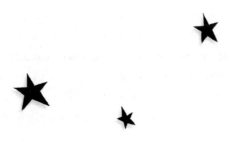

3.

IT ALL STARTS WITH YOU

*One of the most fundamental journeys I have been on over the past decade
is the journey towards a commitment I made to never again put myself
last. It was inspired by a community of women who came into my life
at a time when I was over-committed and exhausted by all my efforts to
support others. Implementing it has been a personal journey as well as a
collective one. I show up better in relationships with others if I've found
time and space for myself. Space to breathe, to sit, to walk, to dance and
to write. These are the practices in my life that deeply nourish me.*

*I had always worked in organisations that were seeking to create social
change. But I have found that if I have practices that nourish and support, I am more actively able to engage in conversations and action that
challenges oppressive systems. One supports the other. And I believe that
a philosophy and practice of care rooted in the collective are the roots of
the tree that can become the change we create in the world. They nourish
it and let it grow over time and allow it to flourish. And if we neglect the
roots, they wither and we struggle, especially in the longer term.*

Mary Ann

Before we dive into how you might create a Red Tent for your community,
we want to talk first about doing this for yourself. This is not because we
think that any of this is really an individual act but rather because we want
to invite you to think about how practices you'll be sharing with others in a
Red Tent operate in your own life. How are they part of how you show up?
How are your ideas and philosophies rooted in your practice, in what you
actually do?

You and Rest and Care

First, we want to invite you to think about intentionally creating spaces in your life in which you can rest and care for yourself.

Perhaps right now you don't have a Red Tent...

Perhaps you can't find one in your area...

Perhaps you are not sure you will make it to one right now with all the other things in your full and stretched life...

Perhaps you are thinking that you might start one but don't feel quite ready yet...?

Wherever you are with this right now, we invite you to practice the principles of care and to think about finding times – moments even – in your day-to-day life in which you can allow yourself to '*be*' rather than '*do*'. To make space for times when you can care for and nurture yourself.

> *You can't pour from an empty cup, you need to take care of yourself... Self care is a ritual for me. I feel you cannot really take care of yourself if you're not making a ritual out of it. And if you're not enjoying it, then you're not nurturing the self. For me it's granting myself the time to be beautiful, to feel beautiful, to just enjoy it.*
>
> **Pascale**

There is also a component of the principles of care which is about building the ability in us to be able to say 'no' to some things we may have filled our lives with, in order to carve out some precious moments for ourselves. As you explore this you might also consider inviting a friend or two to join in and share what you are doing and hold one another accountable.

You can experiment with ways of caring for yourself and for one another. It doesn't need to be complicated. Ask yourself: *what would feel nourishing and replenishing for me today?* And choose to do that – be it going for a walk in the sunshine (or rain!), having a bath if you have one or simply taking ten minutes to put your feet up. We share some more ideas for what you might do a little bit later in this chapter!

First, we want to acknowledge that the capacity we have to take this kind of action in our lives varies greatly. For some women taking any time out at all is impossible. Caring responsibilities for children, parents and others make it more difficult, as can the demands of our work or other activities. The time we have is also significantly affected by our level of privilege and access to money and support. The more marginalised we are in the society in which we live, the more this is likely to be the case and so race, class, access to resources and other factors greatly impact how much space for respite society affords us.

As a working-class person, self-care has always left me full of guilt. I rarely do anything for myself that doesn't also benefit someone else. I don't take breaks or holidays and I rarely buy anything of value that isn't absolutely necessary. I'm not very good at switching off from things as I know that someone somewhere will be needing my attention as soon as I power down.

Kim

One great thing about community-led Red Tents is that they can provide space for women who find it harder to take time and space for themselves because of other responsibilities and restrictions in their lives, especially if a Red Tent can help support women to take a break from childcare and other responsibilities in some way.

My dream scenario would be that the elders or perhaps teenagers of the group take turns in offering childcare for a mother circle, so the group has childcare. I think that would be the best way of doing it. Potentially, it could still even be a mixed group of mothers and babies and, people without babies too. If you provide childcare, it enables women with small children not to be excluded from the Red Tent at a time when they may need it most, but it requires a commitment from those elders to step out of the circle sometimes. That would be my dream setup.

Lily

Through our own experience and that of the many women we have worked with we have found that alongside the very real restrictions in many women's lives many of us have narratives that make taking even small amounts of time for ourselves pretty difficult. It's not just that we don't have time – though many women say this to us, and we have said it to ourselves often too – underneath the lack of time, we have found that there are often many other narratives at play.

We may have a low sense of self-worth that affects our ability to appreciate what we bring to the world and it may be linked to a sense of scarcity more generally. We tell ourselves we will do it when we have just finished 'x' or 'y'. We tell ourselves that we will have time in the holidays, when term starts again, when this project is finished... We tell ourselves we don't deserve it, it's selfish, it's only for other people with nothing better to do.

But we have also found that when we can identify and even perhaps laugh at some of these internal narratives, we begin to realise that it is when we are most overstretched and think we don't have time that we really need to rest. These very dynamics continued to be present for us sometimes in the writing of this book. Changing these stories is a continual process and one which we encourage everyone running a Red Tent to commit to being in the practice of. To commit to being in active enquiry about the rest and replenishment they need, and where they might be depriving themselves of it. In many ways the Red Tent itself, the simple act of taking some space to care for and replenish ourselves flies in the face of cultures that expect us, particularly women, to be-it-all and do-it-all.

As women we do a lot of caring for others. We learn through experience to be good carers, but often it feels like there is no one to care for us. When we sit in a Red Tent circle we sit as equals: we can give, we can receive, we can relax and let the energy flow. It gives me energy to go back out into the busy world and be myself in a more balanced powerful way.

Juliet

Many women feel the pressure directly and indirectly to place a number of things first in their lives such as family, community, work and purpose, and to try to maintain an equally high standard in them all. Our culture also supports this. For example, hard-working women in the spotlight are often criticised for their looks and dress sense whilst men in similar positions seldom receive comments about how they look. Whilst women working in caring professions are praised for their self-sacrifice and wind up working on a day off or when they are clearly sick and need to rest. These are the kinds of expectations we have learnt to accept.

If you want to start a Red Tent in your community, being able to think about these dynamics and practice finding ways to take some space, however small, for yourself first – or in a small group – can help you develop the very things you want to bring into being in a Red Tent space where women can care for themselves and each other. And so being in this practice and enquiry can help you to stay authentic to your vision.

Care Activities you can practice alone or with others

Self-care, a term described by queer, Black feminist, Audre Lorde, as a political "act of self-preservation" has become a fashionable meme and buzzword often associated with things you can buy with money like massages and essential oils. These may be wonderful, but we also believe that we have the resources within us to offer ourselves the basic care and attention we need, to counter the part of us that is ever responding to the constant needs and wants for others. Within us we have the tools that work for us if only we can make the space to find or remember them. Taking time for ourselves in culture that invites us to demonstrate our worth by how much we are able to do and achieve, can be a radical, counter-cultural act. We invite you to think for yourself about how you might commit to practicing the kind of self-care that really works for you and to think also about the collective practices that nourish you. We are thinking about:

* Our breath (just noticing it is a start – while many meditation and mindfulness practices go deeper with this).

* Physical movement (of any type) – we like the kind that makes us feel joy in our bodies rather than the need to 'burn' fat or calories. We might do this alone or in company.

★ Going outside in nature, including looking at the sky, the horizon or the changing weather. Again this might be alone or in company.

★ Finding somewhere private to get a few minutes peace (it can be the toilet – in fact Mary Ann shares with her clients the idea that you can take a brief break in an office environment by going into the toilet with headphones and listening to something relaxing or dancing to something fun!).

★ Making ourselves the food we love and that feels nourishing to us (share it with friends or loved ones or simply treat yourself!)

★ Spend an afternoon in a bookstore or library, just browsing.

★ Take yourself out for the afternoon on a date for one. Use the time to write, read or simply enjoy being. Or spend time with a friend or lover in this way.

★ Give yourself an afternoon off to simply wander. Set out inquisitive but without a plan and see what happens. Again, you might share this practice with someone else.

★ Share what is going on for you right now in the presence of a witness. If you don't have a friend or therapist to do this with, you can also do it alone using a journal or record your voice so you can witness and acknowledge yourself. Choose the things that truly nourish you. Don't be seduced by what is 'meant' to feel good to you. If it doesn't feel good and supportive to you, don't do it.

We are thinking about equipping ourselves as leaders and community holders by honouring our own needs first. Perhaps this may feel selfish for you. Our cultures often teach us that we must meet others' needs first. The result of this is our tiredness and exhaustion which isn't really good for anyone in the longer term.

This isn't about making ourselves the centre of everything, but it is about honouring what we need to be able to show up for others, for the community Red Tent space which we want to create. So we want to invite you to build practices from the very get-go that honour your needs. As you create a space in your Red Tent in which women come together to rest each month how can you make that pausing and honouring of space also a practice in your own life?

In Mary Ann's work she has mapped so many ways in which the people she has worked with find they are expending themselves and see that culture encouraged in the world around them. She often invites the people and organisations she works with to consider what would change if they refused to be expendable? This is a question you can also ask yourself to reflect or journal on as part of your practice.

REFLECTIVE QUESTIONS

✶ What am I truly longing for?

✶ What would feel good to me today?

✶ How can I look after myself better?

✶ What would change if I refused to be expendable?

Care as a Liberatory Act

As we have already alluded to in the previous section, we believe that care for ourselves and each other is the foundation of work that challenges oppressive systems. We have both worked in the NGO space for many years and seen how burnout, self-sacrifice and saviourism can show up and take hold.

And so, when we invite you – through the pages of this book – to commit to making your Red Tent a liberatory and anti-oppressive space, we are not saying exhaust yourself or make yourself a martyr. And that's why we began this chapter with a focus on care. Now we have that straight, we want to invite you to think about building liberatory and anti-oppressive practice as personal and political work. Feminists have long made the assertion that the personal is political. The political idea of patriarchy and the oppression of women is experienced in our personal lives just as much as the other spaces we may move in. And this, of course, includes Red Tent spaces.

And so, whilst we see oppressive systems as structures way beyond each individual who may be participating willingly, ignorantly or unwillingly in them, we also see individual and collective acts of resistance, at a small day-to-day scale. Within Red Tents we see this as part of what can, over time, build the emergent culture that can help to challenge those systems and create cultural and systemic change.

In other words, what we *do* matters as much as what we think and believe. And so the question we want to invite you into is: *how can what you do, both personally and collectively within your life and – if you run or attend one already – your Red Tent too, build a day-to-day practice of anti-oppressive and liberatory action?*

We will continue to talk about what that can look like through the pages of this book, but as we open these questions for you, we wanted to share a few reflections on the personal parts of this practice.

One of the reasons we want care to be our foundation, is that we want to settle our nervous systems and process our own trauma and pain enough that we are able to be in active practice of creating cultural change. This is usually about finding a way to acknowledge what is our stuff and not forcing it down, pushing it away or numbing it out. This is not about being perfectly healed individuals or groups. We are most certainly in the messy middle of this, perhaps you are too?

It is about noticing that when we talk about challenging oppressive systems with actions that are liberatory, feelings and sensations come up in our bodies that may not reflect the reasoning of our rational minds. In other words, our reactions may not be in line with our values. Our instinctive actions may perpetuate oppression without our deliberate agreement. We recommend exploring the work of Resmaa Menakem who demonstrates how addressing racism requires body-based practice and not just an intellectual pursuit. As he puts it, "We've tried to teach our brains to think better about race. But white-body supremacy doesn't live in our thinking brains. It lives and breathes in our bodies." [1]

We think that Red Tents are one of the spaces in our lives where we may be able to encounter the sharing and processing of our experiences. We are also aware that they are spaces where oppression can come up or be replicated and so building our own awareness of this complexity is key. We do not all have the same lived experiences. But being aware of our own and the things that trigger us is an important key in building collectively run and led Red Tents.

Here are some of the thoughts and feelings we have noticed coming up as we try to build liberatory practice:

★ the sense that we are always getting it wrong;

★ the sense that we may be losing something if we change;

★ attachment to the idea that we are 'one of the good ones';

★ experiencing the anger of others as being about us personally, when it may actually relate to a broader oppressive system and the way in which we have embodied it;

★ noticing how many of the voices in the Red Tent community seem to look and sound like us and needing to reach out further to share with a greater diversity of women;

★ feeling uncertain about what we think and what we should do;

★ fear that we will make mistakes and be judged/judge ourselves harshly for them.

1 Menakem, Resmaa. *My Grandmother's Hands: Racialized Trauma and the Pathway to Mending our Hearts and Bodies*

All this is to say that these thoughts and feelings – and likely many others – might come up as you engage with the material in this book and the ideas we are sharing. This is completely normal. As adrienne maree brown says, "We all have work to do. Our work is in the light. We have no perfect moral ground to stand on, shaped as we are by this toxic, complex time. We may not have time, or emotional capacity, to walk each path together. We are all flailing in the unknown at the moment, terrified, stretched beyond ourselves, ashamed, realizing the future is in our hands. We must all do our work. Be accountable and go heal, simultaneously, continuously. It's never too late." [2]

The thing about oppressive systems is that they are deliberately set up to make it hard to challenge or question them. The resilience and success of these pervasive systems is upheld by our complicity with them. And so when we are challenged we often react in line with the system, resisting the idea that we may be at fault, that we may have acted out of unconscious bias. We have to learn to expect resistance to come up in us and then make space within ourselves to challenge our assumptions, rather than reacting immediately to 'stay safe' and maintain the status quo.

What if you could think about your discomfort as a sign of the oppressive system being active in you? For example, when one of us, as a white person, is attached to the idea that we are 'one of the good ones' in relation to racism, what if we could see that as one way in which white supremacy operates in us, always trying to be the best, do the best, know the best? How might that change how we react to and express our own reactions?

We will talk more about this in the rest of this book but for now here are some suggestions for you as you read:

★ go slowly, especially when you notice something is difficult or uncomfortable for you;

★ breathe deeply. Track the sensations in your body. Go outside. Drink water. Let your system settle;

★ have compassion for yourself and where you are at, rather than judging what you are feeling and thinking: 'I should or I shouldn't be feeling this';

2   brown, adrienne maree, *We Will Not Cancel Us – And Other Dreams of Transformative Justice*

⭑ if you are resistant to the content in this book, you might be learning something important or you may also simply disagree with us. It could well be both. We invite you to discern for yourself.

The personal part of the life-long journey of building more liberatory and anti-oppressive practice has everything to do with embracing the discomfort that arises. One way of thinking about it is that oppressive systems make some people comfortable at the expense of others. So, white supremacy makes white people feel comfortable. Patriarchy makes men feel comfortable. Ableism makes people who do not have a disability comfortable. And so on.

If, like us, you are a white woman, then likely white supremacy may be making you feel comfortable, whilst patriarchy oppresses you. It can be confusing. It's also deeply frustrating for Black, Indigenous and people of colour, and particularly women, when in this discomfort white women fall into relying on white supremacy for their comfort. This is, at least in part, what is at play in *white feminism,* a feminism that centres the struggles of only white women and which seems to argue over who holds the power within the current system, rather than highlighting and dismantling the wider inequality it functions by. Similarly this may play out for *spiritual white women* who prioritise the comfort they find in spiritual practices that are very often appropriated, above the need to speak out about and challenge oppressive systems, thereby benefitting from the comfort of white supremacy as they practice traditions that others have been oppressed for.

We don't want any part in that. And so instead we choose the complicated and messy journey of trying to do something different. We hope you'll join us.

REFLECTIVE QUESTIONS

⭑ What challenges you about the idea of liberatory and anti-oppressive practice?

⭑ What is coming up in your body as you read this?

⭑ What practices might support you to care for yourself as you read on?

4.

LIBERATING SPACE

Decolonization requires that we reclaim the ways of our own stories, our own ways of talking. It also requires also that we think beyond concepts like inclusivity. When we say "inclusive," the opposite is also a truth: exclusive. Inclusivity is a word offered like a fruitless olive branch. It does not mean what we want it to mean, but it does mean what too often is intended. Extended as an empty gift, when we say inclusivity we too often mean "if you will take on my cause, we can fight together." Or "let me tell you what the cause is, and you can join the struggle." When I say, "You are invited," I mean the table is already set in my home and you can come if you like. This may be nice for a dinner party, but it is no way to create a coalition.

LaSara Firefox Allen [1]

When we discussed inclusion with women running Red Tents for this book we found that many seemed to be taking it for granted and in so doing, making an assumption that it was present by default. But when we assume that everyone is welcome it can often disguise and obscure the many ways in which how we do things may make the spaces we create uncomfortable or unwelcoming for others, especially others who have a very different lived experiences to us. We may be used to *normal* being a situation where many are excluded unconsciously, and so we are all at different stages of unlearning our various default exclusion biases.

For example, within white supremacy, whiteness tends to dominate and this

1 Allen, LaSara Firefox. *Jailbreaking the Goddess: A Radical Revisioning of Feminist Spirituality*

means that Red Tents, especially if they are created by white women, will usually by default, be most comfortable for them. As a result, women of colour may not feel welcome. Perhaps because there is no one who looks like them in the space. Perhaps because they have not been explicitly welcomed. Perhaps because they sense what they have to share might not be familiar or acceptable. Perhaps because they do not see themselves represented in the Red Tent spaces we create, which are currently overwhelmingly led by white women.

Our vision for Red Tents and for this work is to invite you, our readers, into the idea of thinking about Red Tents as potentially liberatory spaces and challenge these defaults and we would love you to consider this in the creation and holding of your Red Tent. At the same time, whilst we strive to create spaces that liberate, we will make mistakes, we will be imperfect, we will need to apologise, learn, repair and try again. Liberatory spaces are not the norm in our culture. We are inviting you to disrupt the status quo and challenge how things are usually done through your practice and we are also learning and challenging ourselves and each other. We believe that Red Tents can provide a space to explore this paradox.

We can start by getting more comfortable with welcoming that imperfection and the fact that creating liberatory spaces doesn't feel anything like being the 'good' or 'perfect' one. It doesn't give us the right either to constantly look down on or critique everyone else. Instead it is a value we can hold, a vision we can move towards and a practice that we can centre when we create Red Tent spaces. Meanwhile being open about making mistakes helps others to learn from them too.

Red Tents exist within a world in which multiple oppressions operate and as a result some of the women who come to your Red Tent may be experiencing barriers which you have never considered. Committing to creating a liberatory space means asking questions that deliberately seek to help you understand and plan to mitigate against the barriers that others might face in relation to your Red Tent. And it means being open to changing what you do when you learn something new or when you receive feedback. However, rather than feeling embarrassed or ashamed, which is sometimes our first instinctive response, we can choose to learn to embrace new understanding with humility.

We also think that the circle practice, which we describe in more detail later in this book, is one structure you can use to collectively ask questions about inclusion and explore how you can create a space that really welcomes all those in your community who would like to attend. We also think that you can create circles to explore problems that emerge and discuss the challenges of a liberatory approach. Using this approach you can potentially address and repair harm too. We have learnt in this work that we very often have to rethink something we thought we knew.

Red Tent is a place of radical integrity, where I can be myself and know that I am held and loved.
Jodi

In order for what Jodi says about the Red Tent being a place of radical integrity to be true for everyone present, we need to create spaces that are liberatory because most spaces we are used to don't actually feel radical like this. We envision Red Tents as spaces that invite those participating to be a part of a resilient and connected community but in order to make them inclusive by design, there are a number of specific issues that we want to invite you to consider in this section.

First consider, who are you?

There is seldom one identity that defines us, we live at the intersections of different privileges and oppressions. Knowing who we are is a first step. Sharing our stories with one another in a Red Tent space where each woman takes some time to speak about her family of origin, identity and the things that are important to her about who she is, can also be a valuable starting point for building more inclusive practice.

The second step is to think more about others.

In a Red Tent space there are usually ample opportunities to listen. Make listening something you value deeply. In the next few pages we are going to talk about a number of different oppressive systems and how they may impact women in your community. We invite you as you read the pages to come to explore your own assumptions and ask yourself what you may not be seeing and what may be clouding your own vision. At the same time, you may find yourself in one or more of the identities that we explore. And you may agree or disagree with what we have said. We are writing from where we currently are in our own understanding, but that doesn't mean that we are not open to changing our own minds again and again.

We write with, and hope you will read it that way, a humility that allows change to be a possibility without making what is on these pages the only, everlasting truth. We also believe that it is not the *responsibility* of someone who identifies in a certain way to educate us (or you) about how to communicate with them to make them feel seen, welcomed and heard.

For them, you asking endless questions may be a difficult and harmful reminder of how much discrimination they have faced and are still experiencing. It may be painful and traumatic to listen to you learning what has long been self-evident to them through their own lived experience. Even if your intention is to learn, the impact of you expecting them to educate you may well be a feeling of further marginalisation or disconnection.

In order to build more liberatory spaces where all women can feel welcome, we all need to take responsibility for building our awareness, knowing that we will not do so perfectly and that we all have blind spots and things we have failed to think through in the messy tangle of our own assumptions, stereotypes and judgements. In addition, listening to and learning from those with lived experience, not just in your Red Tent spaces but also beyond it, including those who choose to offer teaching or support, is always a valuable part of building your own understanding.

What is Missing? Who is Missing?

The rigour of being liberatory in the way we organise our Red Tents can begin with asking the following questions:

What is missing that needs to be present to create a more liberatory space?

Who is missing from this and needs to be welcomed?

How do we need to broaden our own thinking in order to take account of intersecting barriers and marginalisations that may be operating in our space already?

Exploring these questions is not so much a theory, it's a practice, it's a commitment, it's ensuring that all of the issues we explore here are things you are regularly considering and reflecting on.

I think the real work now is to reach the place that is not comfortable. You know, you see that woman at the bus stop, she looks different from you…and this is why it's going to be powerful…go and reach out and tell her "Hi, I'm doing a woman's circle, would you be interested in coming?" Otherwise you're just replicating the same circle. You're not opening the system. It's a closed loop system.

Pascale

A liberatory space needs to be a place of equity, by which we mean a space where there is commitment to "disrupting the status quo, re-examining and overhauling power dynamics and creating justice."[2] This opens up the possibility of a diversity of perspectives, a celebration of difference and the inclusion of multiple perspectives. This commitment is, we believe, critical to breaking down the false barriers which so often polarise our world. When we say that we have a vision for Red Tents as liberatory spaces, we mean that we think they can be part of creating ways of being together across difference where our differentness can be acknowledged, celebrated and welcomed.

We need to be able to carry this approach through everything we do, so we can act together, without excluding each other or overlooking one another. But standing hand in hand and saying: *You belong and I belong. All of you, all the parts that make up you, are welcome and needed in this space.*

Gender, Identity, and Rights

The idea of inclusivity is not to view cis women as the norm and others as tolerated, but to aim for true inclusion where everyone is included as normality. Otherwise it is (just) token inclusion.

Heidi

2 Desiree Adaway and Jessica Fish, *Diversity & Inclusion Primer 2018* adawaygroup.com

I've seen the effects on young trans girls and women who have been pet-rified they will be rejected or excluded if they sought help in a women's group...I'm horrified anyone would think of turning them away. We can be better than this. It undermines the whole concept of bringing together and creating sisterhood.

Clare

When we first started the Red Tent Directory, we described Red Tents as spaces for women, without much thought about what was implied by, and who was included within that term. Since then we have had a lot of questions come up within communities about the inclusion of trans women and genderqueer people in Red Tents and we have been providing ad hoc support to holders of Tents on this topic. In the process we have learnt a lot from trans women and those who have welcomed them in their Red Tent spaces. They have shown us – wholeheartedly – and we hope that as you read this section they will also show you – that including trans and non-binary people in your Red Tent is an obligation rather than an option.

Firstly, we have learnt that it is culture that makes us a woman rather than our biology, our physical sex. Culture is gendering us in one way or another based on that sex. But it doesn't have to be that way: gender could have been understood by human beings very differently.

Until I met with a trans woman I hadn't thought about the fact that it wasn't just women like me[3] who have this experience of feeling compli-cated about being a woman, because we know our bodies don't perform the things that a woman's body is supposed to do. There are other women who've also got that going on in really different ways. It was really amaz-ing to meet her and talk. I think that's really when I first met proper fem-inist theory and started reading essays by people about what womanhood meant, and learning about the difference between gender and sex, which no one had taught me before. And I think discovering that was really instrumental in figuring out that I didn't have to be defined. It was a

3   When she says 'like me' Lu is referring to her experience as intersex. She was diagnosed with MRKH when she was a teenager.
For information and support see mrkh.org.uk

journey of curiosity and I started getting fascinated about it.
Lu

We now understand gender to be more fluid than we were brought up to believe, and understand trans and non-binary people to be oppressed by the same patriarchal, supremacist system that women more generally struggle with. Red Tents are a form of rest and replenishment from this system. As Persia, who is a trans woman, explains:

I think the division of the people of the world into two simple categories according to their bodies is the beginning of the problem... So the problem that women have is being classified as what they are in terms of their capacity, intelligence, their strengths and all these things is because they have a different body from a male. To just define ourselves by our bodies denies what, in my opinion, is the whole of us... Defining ourselves by our bodies falls into the trap of the gender binary, which is a way that men have used to have control over women. So it seems to me that that's not an advisable way to go.

When we say *women,* we are clear that we are not talking only about cis women. Instead we include all cis, trans, intersex, and non-binary AFAB people. We believe a Red Tent is a place for you and there is a place for you at the Red Tent.

We have also come to understand that it is our patriarchal system that both defines what femaleness is, and, at the same time, relegates those who have so called *feminine* qualities, attributes, ways of being in the world and *femmeness* to a lesser status, the status ascribed also to *women.* In the words of Julia Serano, "For some time, the understanding of liberation beyond gender roles has been to reject the constructs and socialization of what it is to be a woman. [But] I was able to make the case that the wholesale condemning of femininity is one of the more unfortunate missteps in the history of feminism." [4]

4 Serano, Julia. *Whipping Girl: A Transsexual Woman on Sexism and the Scapegoating of Femininity*

Therefore the discussion about the inclusion and exclusion of people who are trans and/or genderqueer often draws on a misogynistic premise that focuses on bodies and their objectification and then uses this to support a binary idea of gender. This same logic is then used to support the exclusion of these women from Red Tent spaces.

One of the issues of the time is that more and more people are going into the non-binary field, which is where they don't really want to be either of these gender binaries. In myself, I live as a woman, as a she in the world, but within me, I think now that I am something outside of the gender binary. I think that it took a long time to get used to this idea. But when I did, I began to see it as a very special blessing. My friend uses the terms 'they' and 'theirs' and when it came to why, it's interesting. They are a lot younger than me and so come into this in a different way, from a different baseline, almost. My friend belongs in a world where there's a lot of young trans non-binary people and several use 'they' a lot more. What they said is that they transitioned when they were about eighteen, expecting and hoping to arrive in this place of being a simple woman in the world, and found out that that didn't happen, which it doesn't. We're always a little different because we're not typical. I use the word typical rather than normal. And so, we arrive in a bit of a different place. And they said, I don't want to actually belong in any of these binaries, because both of them are too limiting, I'll be non-binary and be 'they'.
Persia

If we understand gender as a construct that has us performing and presenting in a certain way some of us may feel strengthened by our gender and others may feel it doesn't fit. What we can hopefully agree on is that whilst it forms a *part* of our identity it's not the whole glorious summary of who we are. What would it be like to take off your gender and allow yourself to feel all of your edges that are squeezed or denied previously when you sit within it?

We know that there are those in the Red Tent community and among women's movements more generally who feel fear and anger about the participation of trans women in women's spaces. But, as we have explained, we believe that this emphasis on biology and a resulting binary mindset is part of the oppressive systems that dehumanise us all, including trans and genderqueer people, and sow division. In many ways non-binary people are rejecting this binary mindset and living into a more liberatory framework of gender.

Meanwhile, we know that violence is a problem in our world and that violence against women, of many different kinds, is endemic.[5] As Laura Bates' most recent book, *Men Who Hate Women*[6] demonstrates there is a frightening proliferation of misogynistic online spaces where sexual violence is encouraged and applauded and in which cis-gendered white men are most active. They are spaces where the narrative, fuelled by the far right, promotes the belief it is legitimate to hate and harm anyone who doesn't look like them.

When we invite you to welcome all those identifying with the gender woman in some way to your Red Tent, we are not denying your experience of sexual abuse or rape or sexual or domestic violence. Nor are we denying our own. We are also not denying these experiences for trans women or those who are non-binary. Violence is a problem for us all.

In my long life it's never been so bad as it [the attack on trans women] is now. It is so organised and it's just so nasty. But you know what, when these stories get repeated, and they press the buttons in women and I feel sometimes that women, understandably, are frightened of male sexuality and violence, because I've had it myself. I know all about this. I've experienced violence and sexual abuse. But the thing is that all of that hatred has been turned towards us. I imagine younger trans women just simply don't want to get involved or have anything to do with this kind of extreme conflict that's going on. Mainly because all we're doing is just trying to get through the day.

Persia

We are holding an awareness of the violence we face and knowing that

5 unwomen.org/en/what-we-do/ending-violence-against-women/facts-and-figures

6 Laura Bates, *Men Who Hate Women: From Incels to Pickup Artists, the Truth about Extreme Misogyny and how it Affects Us All*

welcoming trans women to our Tents does not make us vulnerable, but instead honours the truth that trans women have rights, and that those who live outside of the limited gender positions in society have rights. Those rights include a welcome in spaces for those that are female-of-centre.

By supporting each others' rights we become stronger and more visible, by seeing the layers within the oppressive systems, within a patriarchal supremacy, we can become more vocal. The argument to suggest that trans women pose a threat is both dehumanising and divisive.

Gatekeeping of this nature always comes from a place of privilege, and is usually exercised towards those with less privilege.
Heidi

There is a privilege for cis people in identifying as the gender which they were assigned at birth and so if you are struggling with this, consider whether you might be gatekeeping out of fear, out of a resistance to change, or because you have the comfort and privilege of being in a position to?

As Rebecca Solnit points out, we need to get over the idea that including trans women will somehow mean that men get into women's spaces. Trans women are women and have a right to be a part of women's spaces. We have all experienced marginalisation under patriarchal systems and have some healing to do, to offer and to share. "Trans women pose no threat to cis women, but we pose a threat to them if we make them outcasts... People – many of whom are supposed to be feminists – keep coming up with lurid 'what ifs'. My response to them is: trans women do not pose a threat to cis-gender women, and feminism is a subcategory of human rights advocacy, which means, sorry, you can't be a feminist if you're not for everyone's human rights, notably other women's rights."[7]

And so we invite Red Tents to be offered as places where women can rest and gain respite from the oppression of the patriarchy and the suppression of the so-called feminine in society and in which those attending can give themselves full reign to express all the parts of themselves that are devalued

7   theguardian.com/commentisfree/2020/aug/10/trans-rights-feminist-letter-rebecca-solnit, Rebecca Solnit

in our wider cultures. As Julia Serano says, "In a culture in which femaleness and femininity are on the receiving end of a seemingly endless smear campaign, there is no act more brave – especially for someone assigned a male sex at birth – than embracing one's femme self... My femaleness is so intense that it has overpowered the trillions of lame-ass Y chromosomes that sheepishly hide inside the cells of my body. And my femininity is so relentless that it has survived over thirty years of male socialization and twenty years of testosterone poisoning."[8]

It is our experience that those Red Tents who already have trans women and non-binary individuals attending find this a positive and enriching experience.

So much of my experience in women's circles is about energetic sharing and holding... I learn so much from my trans friends, their magic is mined from a very deep place. Empathy, love and kindness is an endless source and making space for trans women only lifts us all up ultimately. We have seen this in the rising of women's rights and other minority groups being heard which in turn helps others be heard. The more of us who feel safe, released and loved, the more powerful we all become. I feel and experience this daily. My own wounds are made no less by making space for other wounds to heal.
Loose

Red Tents are offered as spaces to explore our lived experiences in the world and how we are finding our place. They are about sharing and learning from each other about parenthood, birth, loss, grief, joy and relationships so that we have a larger understanding of ourselves and each other. We can use terms such as female-of-centre to align Red Tents as a gathering that welcomes and celebrates the feminine expressions of our lives and moments we go through. This makes them more inclusive of non-binary, intersex and non-binary trans people who want to be in spaces that other cis and trans women are in.

---

8   Serano, Julia. *Whipping Girl: A Transsexual Woman on Sexism and the Scapegoating of Femininity*

We have used, till recently, the term non-binary femme to give a guideline marker where we do not really wish to gate-keep with hard and fast rules or draw a line that is harmful or triggering. We realise now that this term may be confusing or perceived as limiting, and are extending it to any non-binary person who feels that their experience encompasses aspects of what is usually framed as the feminine experience, be it through their assigned gender at birth, their gender presentation or their internal sense of their gender. That leads on to where do you draw the line? This we have gone over and over, chatting about the right language to be inclusive, but also to somehow draw a line in the middle of the non-binary spectrum.

Recently we had a non-binary Red Tenter wondering about our use of the term non-binary femme, and asking at what point would they not be welcome? Did we mean non-binary people who feel more feminine than masculine? Or dress more feminine? Then we realised that people's perception of that word 'femme' may make them feel unwelcome, if they didn't understand what we meant by it.

Now our Red Tent aims to balance the recognition of experiences that women and non-binary people share, whilst honouring that these two identities are not the same and that non-binary people, regardless of gender assigned at birth or presentation, are not women unless they say they are.

Heidi

As we learn from Heidi's approach it is essential to keep having these conversations and take a learning approach. This also applies to sexuality as well as gender. Those identifying as cis, trans and non-binary may also see themselves in a range of different ways in relation to their sexuality and so we must be careful not to make assumptions about this. An inclusive and equitable Red Tent welcomes women whether they identify as lesbian, bi-sexual, asexual, pansexual or heterosexual. We can do a lot right now to ensure that Red Tents are liberatory, resilient and inclusive spaces that we believe they can be. So let's look at what we can do to make this clear.

There is no place for discrimination or prejudice in circles which are meant to be and are advertised as healing and welcoming. I often hear Red Tent leaders say they will check with their group how they feel about

having trans women in the group… I don't feel this is an appropriate response or approach.
Clare

★ Be clear about your standpoint but also make space where necessary to discuss trans and non-binary inclusion with your Red Tent. You can use a circle format (see later in the book) to explore any challenges and questions that may come up with this, but ensure that you do this in a way that doesn't cause harm to anyone present. If in doubt, ask individuals whether they would like to be present for a discussion or what support they might need.

★ Agree how to communicate about gender inclusion in your community so that if someone asks you are clear. Have a draft response ready to send out if someone asks for clarification about your trans and non-binary inclusion policy.

I would urge groups to pre-empt the question by already having an answer to hand. I would encourage groups to open their hearts and arms way before a trans woman approaches their circle, so the decision is already a yes.
Heidi

★ Make clear that trans and gender-nonconforming people and those who identify as non-binary know that they are welcome by making it clear on the invitation or event.

In our circles we have always had participants and leaders from the trans and non-binary community and often find it helpful to think … who isn't in the room and why? … I feel we can always do better with this and it's a work in progress but more urgent in these times.
Clare

★ Explore terminology and get clear on what you mean by it so you can clearly explain to people and they can become familiar with using it.

'Feminine' is a word that I have struggled with. And I think if you'd asked me 10 years ago, I'd have been quite anti that word as a gendered stereotype. But I think, actually, I like the definition of feminine and masculine as descriptions for traits and qualities that all people have, in varying quantities and styles, say that I have feminine and masculine energy bits of me. And finding space to reflect on that feels important.

Lu

One of the ways in which women describe Red Tents is that they sometimes call them *feminine* spaces. We haven't used this term much in this book because for us defining what is *feminine* and what is not can still feel problematic. But we also know that there are a range of things that are often *coded as feminine* in our cultures and which we explore and embrace in Red Tent spaces. Sometimes these are also described as femme qualities.

They include the invitation to be supportive of one another, to connect deeply, to share what is in our hearts, to weep and empathise, to replenish and explore, to create beautiful spaces and rituals we can share and to express parts of ourselves that we often have to hide or at least keep less magnified in the rest of our lives.

If we consider that we mostly operate in a linear world dominated by what we might term *masculine* approaches to problem solving, leadership and power, then we can think of Red Tents as a space where we can disrupt and create spaces that celebrate and focus on alternative and so-called *feminine* ways. To use this analogy, this does not mean negating or rejecting our so-called *masculine* parts but perhaps dusting off the *feminine* parts that have been squashed and kicked aside for so long and placing them front and centre to reflect on.

Many Red Tents have described this process as celebrating the *divine feminine,* an immutable quality that is ever-present in each of us whatever our gender and holding it as something precious, sacred and sturdy beyond stereotypes or projections. We like to see the *divine feminine* as the divine nature of all women which emerges in a million different ways as diverse as the lived experiences of women.

As women we are not really encouraged to explore our feminine strengths, however what we are taught to do is how to fit into the male mould. So for that reason I went along to my first Red Tent, as I wanted to really connect and re-awaken my feminine energy. Cliché as it may sound, it has proved to be a magical place which has always given me exactly what I am after, whether that be connection, reflection or silence, it's a space to let go and just be.

Renée

The feeling of arriving home that women often mention when coming to a Red Tent is to us a coming home to a part of ourselves that has been socialised out of our culture and devalued to the point of suppression. Recognising this can feel healing if we have felt unable to fully express these parts of ourselves in our lives, exiled to the *masculine* world or the narrow filter of what is socially acceptable for women to be and do.

For Red Tents to celebrate the female-of-centre space they are creating while making sure that the language is big enough to still feel useful and inclusive is a complex balance. But it is essential for those who feel limited by gendered terms to know that they can rest, heal and recharge in those spaces too.

Our Red Tent has been non-binary inclusive for quite some time. Although it was originally founded to support women and girls, as time went on, and we became aware of gender needs and other issues, we felt that some of our non-binary siblings would also benefit from the support that Red Tent offers because they experience misogyny, patriarchy and challenges due to their presentation or the way the wider world treats them. Some non-binary folk who were assigned female at birth also desire access to the space to be able to chat about, and gain support during the menstrual years, menopause, and pregnancy. While the term non-binary covers many genders, we as a Red Tent are a space to honour the feminine and give those experiencing misogyny as well as the lived realities of menarche, menstruation, pregnancy, childbirth and menopause a space to come together and share.

Heidi

As Red Tent Basel, Switzerland say, "Our Red Tent is a feminist space. Feminist in the sense that a) we want to create a space to empower women from all walks of life and b) we don't view the concepts of 'femininity' and 'masculinity' as a natural given but as social constructs. We prefer to use the plurals of these terms, i.e. 'femininities' and 'masculinities' instead of the singular. By using the plural, we recognise that there are many different ways of living as women and it allows us to talk about our shared and different experiences. This specifically includes experiences of trans women and queer femmes. Our goal is to witness each other, learn from and lift each other up. "

One way to create a more liberatory space is to allow for and encourage people to share their experience, not as one person representing a whole group of voices but just as themselves as they find themselves in that moment: to use the word 'I' rather than 'we' and to really speak from their own lived experience.

What's important is not to just assume that everyone's living their life the way you're living yours.

Lu

As a person holding space and working collectively with others and holding a vision of liberatory space you can also welcome those with different life experience to hold space and lead alongside you. It's also, as Heidi says, about leading by example as well,

I feel that if enough women stood up as good leaders, holding space for cis and trans women, and non-binary femme/AFAB people without fuss or batting an eyelid, and make it the norm, then others would follow. When good space holders create safety and allay everyone's fears, then education by osmosis can happen. For me, if someone chooses not to come to our Red Tent because we have trans women in our circle, then that is fine, we aren't the circle for them. I can only offer what is in my heart to offer, what feels loving and encompassing and right.

Heidi

★ If you are new to learning about genderqueer terminology then it's important to read up and learn about gender identity and expression. This can support you to have a wider understanding of people's lived experiences and anticipate what people may like or not like about a space. It will also help you to receive feedback from a place of learning rather than defensiveness.

As a non-binary person, it has always felt weird being in cis female spaces – be that virtual or physical. I often feel like I don't quite belong and that people probably would rather I wasn't there. I often seek to remind people on Facebook that they ought not address a group as "ladies" unless they are certain the group consists of only ladies. Sometimes I get a warm reception, other times, I get ripped to shreds! I am in a few Facebook groups that are aimed at ladies but welcome non-binary AFAB people but, again, I feel like I don't quite belong.

Kim

We can always get better at holding ourselves accountable and saying sorry when we make a mistake. It is possible to make mistakes with words but still let people know you see them with respect and openness and apologise to make amends. Transparency is the key to making our Red Tent spaces safer and more inclusive of those that choose the pronouns she/her and they/them.

I think much about gender is learnt and internalised throughout our lives, but it is hard to 'shake' the linear connection between girl and woman. It is extremely well entrenched and difficult for people to think about differently. That doesn't mean we shouldn't try, however.

Madeleine

★ Treat everyone who comes to your Red Tent with the same level of attention and care. Sometimes by over-compensating for perceived difference we may emphasise difference unintentionally. It may well still be harmful and uncomfortable for the person being overly pampered or deferred to.

What do I not love? I don't love the expectations placed on me in these spaces. I'm supposed to feel 'honoured' or 'lucky' to be 'allowed' in such sacred spaces. I am expected to simply toe the line and not cause any waves…and I'm not that kind of person at all. I may not be a woman, but I am still read as such and have spent the majority of my life living as such, so I don't owe those who identify as women a damn thing. Especially when many of them would rather I didn't occupy spaces with them.

Kim

★ Find ways to include in your introduction at the Red Tent some of the key principles of your group. We like what Persia held as her vision for us: "We need to have safer spaces for all people who have been oppressed by their gender. We, all of us, want the same things. Safety for what and who we are is at the foundation of everything we do. A place where we all find respect, recognition and love for who we are."

★ Allow all those who come to feel free to share what they want to. Do not assume that a non-binary person will always want to share about their identity.

★ Remember that it isn't the responsibility of every non-binary or trans person to educate you about their identity and lived experience.

★ If someone is nervous about attending a Red Tent then they may appreciate having a more extensive explanation about the process and way of doing things in the group – "This happens and then we do this…"

When we talk about safe spaces what we are talking about is safer spaces created by the parameters that we put in place. This is integral to Red Tents as we want everyone to show up and feel able to receive what they need. That is why we create structure, talk about ways of behaving, hold ourselves with compassion and invite others to do the same. By having gentle ways to hold us as we meet in a Red Tent we can open our ears and our eyes.

Aisha

We invite you to explore this section and your own practice and at the same time to be aware that you may currently have trans and non-binary people at your Red Tent and not know this aspect of their identity. The invitation is to learn and, where necessary, change. This includes thinking about how you will respond before you receive enquiries from trans and non-binary people. The burden of oppression is very real and very scary for those who are directly targeted and for their parents, caregivers, and friends. So we invite all those who attend or organise Red Tents to go one step further and speak up about ways that trans or non-binary people are criticised, objectified, dehumanised, criminalised, scapegoated, judged, demeaned and attacked. [9]

Right now, transgender women are one of the most at-risk groups of people out there. My group has always been open to transgender women, and always will be.
Ruby

Racial Justice and Anti-Racist Practice

We live in the context of white supremacy, by which we mean that being raced as white in our cultures at this time has afforded those of us who are – including both of us – significant privileges and advantages, many of which we have not always been aware of. We grow every day in awareness of our own privilege. Creating a liberatory space necessitates creating a space that is actively anti-racist and that is playing a role in imagining new ways to relate to one another that are not rooted in a racialised hierarchy.

Whilst white women may experience other forms of marginalisation, we live in the context of having been afforded that privilege at the expense of others and this means that whatever other challenges we may have experienced, those of us raced as white do not experience racism. We do not experience discrimination based solely on the colour of our skin. We are not judged the minute we enter a room or walk by someone on the street on that basis. Racism has not and will not impact everything about our lives.

9   We would like to extend our thanks to Laverne Cox for expressing this so clearly in her film *Disclosure*

And so we have to choose actively anti-racist practice. It is not a necessity for us, because white supremacy protects us, and allows us to stay comfortable without challenging it. But we do have a choice. We can choose to take action, speak up and let at least some of the comfort of that protection go.

Many Red Tent spaces have been initiated by white women and are attended mostly by them also. We know that this is not exclusively true and we interviewed some women of colour who run and attend Red Tents for this book. But given the current context of many Red Tents being white majority spaces, we want to invite all Red Tents to explore anti-racist practice.

I think that people often gravitate to what feels comfortable for them. Like, it must be okay, because it feels right. But I think what we're talking about is: it must be important, because it feels hard, you know, it feels uncomfortable or awkward. Don't shy away from those interactions just because you don't feel so comfortable in them…get to know yourself at your edges.
Aisha

Anti-racism is not simply about having a policy of welcoming or inviting women of colour to your Red Tent. It is about creating a space in which, if and when they come, they might feel welcome. It is about creating a space in which unlearning all the ways in which we embody racism can happen. This is not simple work. It is not a quick fix. Centuries of pain and trauma cannot be erased in one Red Tent meeting. But taking individual and collective steps to be part of the healing rather than perpetuating the problem is possible.

I have often heard it said in a kind of New Age cliché that "whoever is in the room are the right people". I think whoever is in the room are the people that our circle advertised to or who saw the flyer or ad and felt it applied to them … I feel we can always do better with this and it's a work in progress but more urgent in these times…
Clare

We have heard it said, more than once, in response to inviting these reflections, that those who come to a Red Tent have been called to come there and that has nothing to do with race. That there is divine guidance in some way and that if only white people show up, that's how it was meant to be. That's what is known as spiritual white-washing where notions of divine guidance or spirituality are used to cover up the actual functions of white privilege and supremacy in the world. Let's be clear: their sole function is exclusion, to make us feel that white people are better, more worthy and yes, perhaps you have thought it, in some way more divinely guided.

That's the very logic behind colonisation: *We know better. Let's take these lands for ourselves. Profit from them. Enslave, kill, rape and impoverish their people. We were divinely guided to do it. To bring them our religion, our knowledge, our way of life. To take them over and have power over them and call them our own.*

And so, anytime you find yourself resisting this conversation, we invite you to consider exploring how white supremacy and privilege are showing up in you, how you might be embodying them. How these fundamental tenets of supremacy and colonisation live in you, explicitly and implicitly, by design or by accident. We know this doesn't always feel easy. It is a daily practice of unlearning and challenging ourselves that we also practice – and sometimes struggle with – for ourselves. The white supremacist in us loves certainty, just as it loves binaries. It loves to know all the answers and get it right. That's how these systems reward us. And so we are also learning to be uncertain, to not be sure.

There isn't a tick box list for this. It is not simply a matter of welcoming people who don't look like you. It takes realising all the ways in which we may not be taking the impact of racism into account. It takes learning as we go. For us anti-racism is a life-long journey and one in which it has been important to learn to see how we are complicit – even when we don't realise it – in a racialised society – and practice making changes and taking action to repair harm.

Mary Ann

At the same time, any discomfort a white person might feel, does not and cannot ever compare to the daily constant burden and harm of experiencing racism. Our responsibility is to welcome our discomfort and use it to help us transform. In our experience this requires the openness to both personal and collective change that we have already spoken about, a willingness to let go and feel like we are losing things (be that righteousness, decision-making power or access to wealth and resources). Instead of striving to be 'one of the good ones' or to be right, we are learning to orientate to change, to call for it and to allow that to be a consistent part of how we live.

The model of the Red Tent, particularly a collectively-held and inclusive model like the one we explore in this book, can, we think, be an environment in which we actively practice anti-racism but, as we hope we have explained here, this takes a commitment to an active anti-racist practice. So what are some ways that you can help build an anti-racist culture?

★ You can start by learning for yourself more about how racism and white supremacy show up in the world if you don't feel well-informed enough already. There are many resources at the end of this book that can help you to do that and many more that you can find online. There's no excuse not to learn more and educate yourself.

★ In the context of Red Tents, it means that we reject the ways in which we come to realise we may be embodying white supremacy and change our practice, building new habits, daring to do things differently. This might include considering how you promote and communicate about your Tent, and about who is welcome. This might involve dismantling your own assumptions about what you do as part of a Red Tent and what you offer to those coming.

★ It could also include inviting diverse women into the leadership of your Red Tent, setting the intention that it will not be a white or white-only led space.

★ Become more conscious of how racism may impact who attends your Red Tent, who feels comfortable there, how you communicate about it. Who are you signalling is welcome? Who might feel more excluded? Does the language you use, images you've chosen and the way you present your Tent appeal more to white women? Is there implicit bias in how you have been presenting it?

★ The model of the Red Tent, particularly a collectively-held and inclusive model like the one we explore in this book, can, we think, be an environment in which we actively practice anti-racism but, as we hope we have explained here, this takes a commitment to an active anti-racist practice.

★ If you decide to have conversations about racism and anti-racism within your Red Tent consider that for white women talking about racism and what they are learning about it can often be a trigger and a cause of distress to those of colour who may be present. Our unlearning can be messy and therefore frustrating and harmful.

★ And so remember that if you spend time during a Red Tent explicitly talking about racism, you need to be clear that building anti-racist practice necessitates people growing an awareness not just of their own feelings, reactions and thoughts about this issue but also of the impact they may have on others. In particular, for a person of colour who has experienced racism their whole life the impact of white women sharing their newly found shock, anger or grief about racism can be an intense reminder of the problem.

As we take on this work and commit to it, mistakes will happen. We will realise that we said the wrong thing. We created a space that felt uncomfortable to someone. We asked something inappropriate or implied something that caused harm. We will see that an action or a word embodied racism, enacted white supremacy. In a small way or a bigger one we will experience moments when we recognise that we are part of the problem. Admitting we are part of the problem is actually the first step. It is brave and fundamental to creating change.
Mary Ann

★ Learn how to admit your mistakes, simply and honestly: "I am sorry. I see how I embodied racism or white supremacy in what I did. I will take responsibility for making amends. I will do my own work without burdening you." And learn to make amends where necessary, to right a wrong, even one that may seem small. This may be scary. Every bone in your body may prefer to hide from your mistake and pretend that it didn't happen, that it wasn't your fault, that you are 'one of the good ones'. But these small actions of making amends and trying to do better are the small pieces of a massive jigsaw. White supremacy cannot fall if we all hide our mistakes and it cannot fall if we continue to avoid putting them right.

The Tent that we held with the focus on anti-racism went well enough, but it was also complicated. Our Red Tent is overwhelmingly white and though I wanted to open up the group to discuss their feelings around our current awakening, I was anxious that a woman of colour would pop on the Zoom only to find a group of white women unloading their feelings about the subject, which might be traumatizing. I've been part of explicitly anti-racist white spaces and the point of them is to unpack and unlearn our racism (and then take action against it) while not subjecting people of colour to our fumbling around. Our Red Tent isn't explicitly a space for white women, but it ends up being that way. I was very aware that we were on shaky ground.

However, it also felt extremely irresponsible not to address the moment [of the Black Lives Matter protests], as white people need to address racism in all the spaces they inhabit. I came cross this podcast which was an interview with somatic therapist Resmaa Menakem who works with white bodies and bodies of culture[10] to understand how the trauma of racism, both when your ancestors experienced it or enacted it, is felt in the body. This felt like an appropriate starting point for us because our Red Tent is very focused on embodiment – one of the founders is a somatic therapist herself.

So, I suggested this podcast to listen to before the Tent, and then during the Tent I led the group in a meditation where they spoke to an ancestor and a descendent – the hope being that the women would leave the Tent with a sense of understanding their place in the world and in history. After that we did our usual circle-share, where we share what is in our hearts, which may or may not have included the present moment and Black Lives Matter.

Natalie

---

10 "On Being with Krista Tippett" Podcast with Resmaa Menakem, 'Notice the Rage; Notice the Silence' June 2020, onbeing.org/programs/resmaa-menakem-notice-the-rage-notice-the-silence/

★ However you begin to do this, it may well feel uncomfortable. We suggest you take your time holding the paradox that whilst there is an urgency to ending white supremacy, being in a hurry to fix everything is also a familiar characteristic of white supremacy culture.[11] Depending on who attends your Tent and how much conversation you have had about these issues before, you may need time to think about how to build anti-racist practice within your Red Tent. You can do this as a collective, perhaps learning together and even starting with those who hold the space first. There's no perfect way but we must all try.

We think anti-racist practice is something we all need to build and that it needs to become part and parcel of the spaces we create and share together, a central component to our Red Tent spaces.

But there are many pitfalls and challenges to doing this well.

★ When you do feel ready to share conversations about anti-racism within your Red Tent you can frame this by reminding people that while Red Tents are a space to share what is in our hearts and minds we can also use discernment to decide what to share when and how. Invite those sharing to think about the impact of what we share about racism on others. When we know we have a position of privilege, the most radical thing to do can sometimes be to limit what we share about an issue like racism and to save our gut honesty for another space. How can we practice listening most to those who have a different experience? How might we centre the voices of those with lived experience of racism if they are present within the space? The invitation to share what is true for us does not negate our responsibility to care for others, and sometimes that means choosing carefully what it is appropriate to share at a given space and time.

As Natalie did, you might want to bring some somatic awareness to this piece also, inviting those present to notice the feelings and sensations that arise when they share and hear one another on this topic. *My Grandmother's*

---

11 You can explore these ideas more in this description of 'White Supremacy Culture' by Kenneth Jones and Tema Okun from *Dismantling Racism: A Workbook for Social Change* which you can read about here: cwsworkshop.org/PARC_site_B/dr-culture.html

hands by Resmaa Menakem [12] has many body-based practices that could support you with this.

★ Be aware that conversations about racism within your Red Tent may bring up difficult dynamics. Not everyone is ready to consider how they embody racism, and not every person who experiences racism wants to talk about it. Conversations about racism in mixed groups may be particularly triggering for some Black and brown people further compounding their sense of isolation and marginalisation.

★ When thinking about how to create a safer space within your Red Tent for everyone, you may need to consider doing some of this work outside of the main Red Tent space.

★ Remember that within a term like 'people of colour' is a huge range of diversity of heritage, background, identity and so on. Terms like these whilst we may find them useful in describing how racism operates can function also to erase the depth and richness of experience and to define everyone as 'other' to whiteness. We suggest using it sparingly. When possible listen to how individuals identify themselves and follow their lead.

We all have feminine, masculine, and more within us. However, our history and our present reality is home to incredible oppression, violence, and trauma, which people of colour, cis women, and members of the LGBTQ+ community are particularly harmed by. We cannot go in a flash from this glaring imbalance to perfect harmony in which all is forgiven. That would be a terrible erasure of the pain and violation of millions of people. We need dedicated spaces which are safe physically and emotionally for these groups.
Ruby

★ Depending on who attends your Red Tent you may need or want to create spaces outside your main Red Tent gatherings. If you are Black,

12 Menakem, Resmaa, *My Grandmother's Hands: Racialized Trauma and the Pathway to Mending our Hearts and Bodies*

Indigenous or a person of colour you might want to create Red Tents that are dedicated spaces for healing and connection of women of colour. These might be spaces to share experiences of racism and heal together and are sometimes described as cohort or caucused spaces, or affinity groups. You could also create spaces in which white women explore their own biases and learn to do better. Or you might create mixed spaces. But be very clear about the content you plan to discuss and offer people options to leave the space and get support if they find them triggering.

★ Be aware that there are people unsure of where and whether they fit in a group described as being for 'people of colour' and 'white' people. Those who are mixed might feel comfortable for different reasons in both spaces. Sometimes they could be described as 'white passing' meaning that whilst they hold a mixed identity, they appear white. These questions are often a space for rich conversation around the things that both divide and unite us. Invite people to choose for themselves. Watch out, however, for white people denying their privilege and trying to explain it away or using the idea that they don't 'feel white' as a way to avoid talking about racism. We can acknowledge that whiteness is not the only facet of our identity and still remain conscious of how it functions in our world. [13]

★ Perhaps you may be able to access other anti-racist practice spaces in your community as a means to learn and think about how to develop your practice within your Red Tent.

I really want to make Red Tents more inclusive. I think it is really important to open up to different types of women. You know, it's just important. The world is changing. Everything is changing. So should the Red Tent. And this is what Red Tents can provide, this surrendering. It is much more possible because you're doing the collective healing. And it's always easier to do it as a collective.

Pascale

13 Mary Ann is a Co-Director of a multi-racial project, Healing Solidarity, that offers healing spaces to people working in international development and so some of this learning comes from their work, which you can find at healingsolidarity.org

To be clear, though this may be challenging, we don't think it is possible to avoid it. If you avoid the issues of white supremacy and racism within your Tent, you are almost certainly going to find yourself complicit in perpetuating them. And this means that unravelling them together is the only way to a more liberatory space in your Red Tent and more broadly in our lives and collective future.

Intergenerational Red Tents

Our Tent is quite intergenerational. I'd say it would range from 18 to 75. I love that. That's one of the best things about the Red Tent for me. It's sitting in circle with older women. And maybe some of the younger women see me as an older woman! Some of these women are so wise... some of those 18-year-olds.
Mads

Whilst many Red Tents run events for specific age-groups such a girls' work or work for older or post-menopausal women, community-level Red Tents often thrive because of the sharing that happens across age groups.

From the point of view of inclusion, awareness about age and the presence of women at different stages of their lives in Red Tent spaces, means being aware that we don't all experience the various stages of our lives in the same way. For example, where some may rejoice in getting older, others may find it a scary or difficult experience.

The wisdom of older women helps younger women to understand life in another way, with less drama and more clearly. It helps young women to feel integrated and confident. It is essential to me that the ages are different so that the whole experience is richer.
Susana

Being intergenerational also means holding an awareness of the issues that may come up around puberty, in the middle of life, during and after-menopause, alongside childbirth and parenting, and all the spaces in-between within Red Tent spaces. Many who have attended Red Tents share that the diversity of ages and lived experiences provide something unique for everyone to benefit from.

The Red Tent is a place where women of all ages come together and tell their stories without being judged. They can support each other in the different phases of their life and experience the powerful energy they can create together.

Kerstin

How might different age groups communicate differently? Consider this when you think about your communications.

Are there ways in which you can reach those who communicate more – or more effectively – in a different way from you?

Do some women still prefer offline communication? Might you reach younger women more effectively in digital spaces?

How do we unpack our welcome so those present feel they will be seen and heard regardless of their age?

Defining the detail

Many Red Tents say that women and girls are welcome, so it makes sense ahead of any enquiries to consider the age of girls welcome into your space. Are girls welcome at any age or only once they reach a specific age? If a few younger women are interested might you be open to setting up of an age-specific group for them? If you do set up a dedicated girls' group you might want to think about how you define the word 'girls' to make it inclusive for young people reflecting on their gender and identity?

Babes in arms

Many Tents welcome 'babes in arms'. It's worth agreeing exactly what this means, i.e. how old is a 'babe in arms'? Many Tents welcome, for example, babies under the age of one. Are there ways that additional support can be provided to mitigate any disruption babies might cause? Whilst we love the welcome of little ones in Red Tent spaces, many Red Tents have found that being very clear about this becomes important if any questions or confusion arise around this issue.

Caring responsibilities

Might you decide to welcome children into your main Red Tent space? For some women who have their own or caring responsibilities for children it can be a challenge to be able to attend Red Tents for what can feel like a substantial period of the young children's life.

I felt isolated as a single mum first, I was thinking wherever I want to go, like in terms of Red Tents, and I cannot make it because kids are not allowed. So I need to make my own Red Tent and allow mums to come with children. It all started like that. But it also started with a feeling of loneliness, feeling like as a mother, you know, I feel very lonely. And I would like to meet other mums or single mums ideally, so we can share our struggles and the joys.

Pascale

Many women of varying ages have responsibilities as carers. Are there ways in which you can take these into account? Can you think about childcare provision or rotating that within your Red Tent so that, even if you aren't able to welcome children of all ages, women can take turns in attending? These structures may be particularly important to enable your Tent to welcome single parents who may have additional childcare responsibilities and needs. If women are caring for older relatives or children with complex needs then having Red Tents that meet during the hours when they have relief support might help them to attend. This can often be around mealtimes or the beginning and end of the day.

Additional Tents

As well as being aware of intergenerational needs, the breadth of ages in your Tent may help you offer additional 'spin-off' Tents to specific age groups perhaps focused on sharing about specific themes. A number of Red Tents have created these circles as an additional resource for women in their community. For example, many groups run girls' circles for girls navigating puberty or 'silver' circles (for elder women) providing collective understanding and support for women who are post-menopausal. Some have also created Parent and Baby Red Tents as a space where women with young children can meet and share, to further meet this need. Girls' groups require some additional or augmented support and are often run with the support and facilitation of an adult.

In a typical session we will sing a song at the beginning which welcomes each girl into the circle. We use a personal talking stick (covered in ribbons, one for each girl taking part) and share our news, lighting a candle as we go round. We introduce a theme for example, if the meeting falls on Valentine's Day it might be about self-love. We will incorporate movement practice. There is often time to share in twos, weaving in the theme, followed by another circle that we all share together. We will anchor this with a craft activity such as making a heart. The girls also spend time in nature together or sometimes alone in a special spot. We round the session off with a song and some snacks to share.

Many of the girls have expressed their excitement of looking forward to their bleeding time. In this community the girls are celebrated as they move up with peers from Moon Daughters to form the next circle. The vision is for the girls to stay together throughout their teenage years. Menarche ceremonies are naturally integrated into the journey of circle life. The monthly moon circles are led by mothers taking it in turn to lead the sessions and supported by mentors who support the girls at gatherings and camps.

Kesty

Understanding some of the challenges for mothers and parents has led to specific Red Tents to support them to meet and have some shared connection with or without the small people being present.

I am so grateful to have witnessed so much, so many stories, feelings, experiences, including my own. We all have something to share, we all have times of feeling the need to be held, seen, nurtured and witnessed. I have learnt not to fix, over-mother or heal. But to trust in the process of being:

being present, being here now knowing that unconditional love is the only way. So many women are deeply tired, mothers are deeply stressed and stretched with a lack of support, unable to ask for help or knowing who to ask where and when. Our society does not value or honour mothers and mothering, and as we all know the power of women has been eroded and snuffed out in our patriarchal culture.

Angie

Where many women appreciate the diversity of ages coming together, others feel there is a need to have their own experience reflected and explored. The benefit of having a place for older women to go to feel visible and empowered in a society that focuses resources and attention on youth can be powerful.

I began to experience a gap in terms of personal life experiences, along with the health challenges that come with age, life cycle changes and body maturation and in some cases being grandmothers (or not). I missed seeing a quiet empathic understanding and nodding of acknowledgment, which comes with the recognition of, "Mmm yeah...I've been there...I get what you are going through". And thus, an idea began to percolate...of setting up a group for us women of 50 plus years. A gathering of women, coming together to share, nurture and acknowledge our challenges and our unique journeys and exchange healing touch, meditation, ritual, movement, poems and songs, loving and celebrating each other.

Reana

Disability and Inclusion

According to a social model of disability – which is what we invite you to adopt – disability is a result of a society that does not fully include people with a wide range of abilities – rather than a consequence of what others might see as something 'different' about a disabled person. A liberatory space is a space in which disabilities are welcomed, recognised and supported as needs just like any other. They are spaces in which inclusion and accessibility become a practice.

If you take this perspective, including people who have a disability is about doing all you can to reverse the ways in which the environment in and around your Red Tent may inhibit their full participation and inclusion. Be sensitive to confidentiality about sharing information to meet needs and holding clear boundaries to protect privacy where appropriate. It is important also to remember that many people's challenges are "invisible" at first glance, including many neurodivergences such as autism, dyslexia, dyspraxia, ADHD, as well as visual and auditory processing issues.

Consider being ready to share with anyone wanting to join your group what support with accessibility you are able to offer. Share as widely as you can what support for this may be available.

Having a welcome person at the Tent that helps people to get comfortable and find what they need can be a great support here.

Communication and Information

With communications clarity and readability is key. Think about the accessibility of information, the online information and anything written that you are sharing. Provide clear instructions and, where possible, maps for reaching the venue. Consider how someone with visual or reading challenges would access the information, for example.

Be clear also about the length of your gathering – this can be especially important for those with sensory issues and those who experience anxiety. Provide a clear description on what the timings include and which aspects are optional (if any).

Physical Accessibility

We live in a society that often presents multiple barriers to people with physical disabilities. How can you create a workable solution in advance if a Red Tent is happening in your home or in another inaccessible or unequipped space? Clarity on physical arrangements is key. Some Red Tents run at venues that do not have full physical accessibility. The first step is to get clear.

Our Red Tent is far from ideal in terms of accessibility because it is upstairs, which concerns me. So far it has not been an issue, but I am not sure how we would resolve it if someone did want to come who could not

manage the stairs. I would always try my best to accommodate.
Jessica

If physical accessibility is a challenge you might consider using community spaces that would provide better provision for some types of accessibility, such as a wheelchair ramp, lift or disabled parking, and be relatively low cost to hire.

Have a plan in place about what arrangements you could offer if someone wanted to come who was unable to access your current venue. That way, it is not the responsibility of the person wanting to attend to find the solutions, you are accountable for that instead. You can make clear in your invitation about the limitations for accessibility but that you have a plan to adapt where necessary. In this way you can acknowledge the issue and also indicate that you want to find a way to resolve it. This communicates your Red Tent is welcoming to people of all abilities, as you hold the responsibility for changing the set up.

It is not just access to the venue that requires consideration, but also sitting arrangements inside: is there an alternative, for example, to sitting on the floor which may be impossible for those with mobility challenges and chronic pain conditions? Lighting can be a big issue for those on the autism spectrum, those with sensory processing issues and for people who experience migraines. If possible, ensure non-fluorescent lighting.

Consider how you can support accessibility in other ways. Are there supports you can provide including working with carers or assistants to facilitate attendance at your Red Tent? Can you offer support with transport also?

Consider those with visual and hearing impairments. In what ways might you help them be able to fully participate in your Red Tent and access the information they may need to do so?

Consider a range of health needs relating to rest needed, medication impacts and concentration spans that people attending your Red Tent might face.

How can you become more aware of accessibility for those on the autistic spectrum? How might visual support materials and clear social guidelines help?

Consider sharing a picture of the room, some of the key women and the entrance way, as well as a clear map on your website or social media.

The opportunities here include developing an understanding of a variety of needs and practically and creatively meeting them. Modelling inclusive space, rather than waiting for an opportunity to create inclusive space, is important in a society that in general disables people rather than accommodates and includes them. *How can you more effectively model an accessible society within your Red Tent?*

Mental Health

Red Tents are like balm for the edges of me that become bashed and bruised by life. In the deep holding space of the Red Tent I remember that all is well and I have sisters who I am connected to across the planet and that feels really important.

Steph

Red Tents are valuable spaces for many women to support their mental health. There are a huge range of issues and diagnoses that can be grouped under this title. Many of us will experience some kind of mental health issue in our lifetimes, by which we mean a whole range of conditions including anxiety, depression, self-harm, and feeling any number of symptoms of being overwhelmed. Others will be managing life-long mental health issues or for those that menstruate there may be times within their monthly cycle where their mental health issues may be amplified. Women will likely share about mental health issues at some point in the sharing parts of your Red Tent.

I was having a miserable second pregnancy fraught with sickness, depression and pelvic girdle pain. Whilst searching for emotional support I discovered Bournemouth Red Tent. Having a space where I could unleash all the feelings and pain I was experiencing without anyone judging me for my ingratitude was exactly what I needed.

Rebecca

A lot can happen in each woman's life and – let's be honest here – life can throw us some pretty tough things to deal with. Women's mental health is also disproportionately affected by a patriarchal society which undervalues women's time, underfunds women's services and undermines women's rights. It is little wonder that women's mental health and wellbeing is such a huge issue and that mental health problems are a common experience.

Please bear in mind that a Red Tent that is collectively led is not and cannot be a professional therapeutic space. Red Tents allow you to be where you are at: you are not going to have your feelings negated, you are not going to be fixed, you are not going to be offered solutions, you are not going to be judged for not knowing the answers to your particular puzzle.

But they are deliberately a community of women, not a professionally facilitated process or means of support. Red Tents have needed, at times, to point this out to those participating so it is worth being clear about this. You might also find yourself suggesting or referring women to other forms of support if women attending do need to request additional support. Although Red Tents cannot replace the value of regular therapy or professional help they can offer a place to be heard, and seen, and welcomed wholeheartedly.

Finding quiet and rest can be challenging when you have constant noise in your head, which is how I experience my own anxiety and depression. For me it is often like a meteor storm of negative thoughts and I barely know which way is up. I think that if you have depression or anxiety you are incredibly brave for choosing to seek company rather than hide, nourish rather than grind yourself through another day, and sit still instead of doing everything to outrun your thoughts. But quite honestly the stopping is the rest in itself, it doesn't need to be anything more than pausing in the company of others. Whether you feel alone or connected, you are disrupting the thoughts that keep you separate. That in itself is an act of courage.
Aisha

As Red Tents often involve unstructured time, those with mental health challenges may find knowing in advance exactly what will happen during a Red Tent gathering particularly important. Many may be managing anxiety or other challenges in relation to attending the Tent. Being clear about what will happen at the Red Tent, in terms of process, may help to allay their concerns. It may be appropriate in some cases to meet with women in advance of a Red Tent to help provide more clarity and support them with any anxiety they may be facing about attending.

Class and Access to Resources

Our level of wealth and that of those around us and with whom we are in community can influence who we invite to our Red Tent, who feels comfortable there and who has access to the space or not. But we can also choose to name these boundaries and challenge them in a number of different ways. A liberatory space welcomes everyone regardless of their ability to pay, which is one of the reasons that a free or donation model is so important to us. We will talk more about resourcing your Red Tent later in the book. It's also worth saying that those with access to more resources can always be invited quietly to donate more and support the group out of an awareness of their own privileged access to wealth. Out of solidarity and a belief in equity rather than out of an inflated sense of their own charity. We like this definition from a resource from the Catalyst Project, "We understand class as a system of power based on perceived and actual social and economic status. In other words, it's a combination of how much access you have to power and money, which determines life outcomes ranging from health, housing, work, and education to how long you live. It also strongly shapes our values, beliefs, and expectations, which deeply inform our ways of thinking and acting throughout life. Capitalism keeps us confused about class and ashamed or afraid to talk about it, which invisibilizes the massive wealth disparity in this country and the systems that keep it in place." [14]

Our silence about class only benefits those with more wealth. But it's something that impacts your circumstances in life and, as we mentioned much earlier in the book, will influence how easy – or not – it is for you to take time for yourself or to have the ability to attend a Red Tent gathering.

An awareness about class and wealth – and analysis of it in relation to your Red Tent – is about helping break down some of the barriers that might prevent people from accessing your Red Tent. It's about having an awareness

14 Definition taken from this resource by the Catalyst Collective: collectiveliberation.org/wp-conTent/uploads/2018/10/Deconstructing-Class.pdf

also of the assumptions you are making that relate to your own 'class' and what might be possible for you as a result of it?

How does someone find out about it [Red Tent]? If it's from someone you know, then how do you know that person? It's probably because you hang around in the same places. And so it just perpetuates that sameness. That is why I think things like having it in the community centre, and advertising it in the local paper or on the coffee shop noticeboards is a really good way of trying to not create an echo chamber.
Lily

Here are some ways to challenge class hierarchies in your communication about your Red Tent:

✶ share leaflets or posters in cross-class venues such as cafés, libraries, doctors' surgeries and community centres;

✶ speak widely about Red Tents so that word of mouth touches women in all your networks;

✶ provide information about public transport links, not just parking provision;

✶ use clear language rather than jargon.

Assuming that you are not charging for your Red Tent, financial barriers are limited. As you will read later in this book, we advocate for a donation-based model. These can be on a sliding scale where those with additional resources can give more to help support the whole Tent. Making communication about money transparent is important as well so that new people have the information and don't feel uncomfortable about financial issues that have not been fully explained.

Consider the timing of the event. How will the timing you have planned impact those who rely on public transport or who do shift work?

How can you think about the provision of childcare in a collective way?

If you want to share your Red Tent with those from different backgrounds to you, you might think about holding an informal gathering in a space that might be unusual to you – but that might be a place where other women gather. Or you might do this within another shared space such as a work-place or community venue or event. This can be a way to gently create space to connect with different women and build links to new audiences. The informal gathering could be a space to share something about your Tent and invite others to join it.

Myself and another founding member came up with the Red Tent Social to try to make our Red Tent more accessible. My house is a distance from central Swansea and we're aware that going to a stranger's house, whom you have only spoken to via the Internet, can be quite intimidating. The Red Tent Social is in addition to our monthly Red Tent, where we meet again in a public venue (pub, park, cafe, etc) just to get to know each other and discuss plans for the next actual Red Tent.
Michelle

Language

Have you thought about what other languages women in your community might use or feel more comfortable with? On the Red Tent Directory we list a number of multi-lingual Tents and so wanted to provide a brief note on this type of accessibility too.

If you decide to be a multi-lingual Red Tent – perhaps because you are based in a location where multiple languages are spoken – you will need to consider whether you have a translation facility or perhaps hold Red Tents in different languages on different days or at different times? It may be more appropriate for someone to share in their language of birth if they want to say something vulnerable and hear themselves say it. This may be the case even if no one present understands their language. Sometimes we can understand much of what is shared through emotion and expression alone without needing actual translation. However, if there are a number of shar-ings in another language it may affect the flow and sense of connection if there is not a *way in* to understanding. Your approach here will need to be nuanced to your own context. There are some Tents where two languages are spoken throughout. If your Red Tent is multi-lingual, you'll need to share publicity in both – or many – languages.

Online Accessibility

Online Red Tents, which became more widespread during the Covid-19 pandemic, can also make Red Tents more accessible to those who struggle to attend in person. This might include those who have caring responsibilities and find it difficult to take time out or those who are ill or recuperating.

They can also be more accessible for those with transport issues or who may not feel safe leaving home, especially in the evening. Those on the autistic spectrum or with anxiety issues might find online spaces far easier to show up to than an in-person meeting…but may also find the amount of information and interruptions overwhelming.

Some simple guidelines can help make online spaces more comfortable and accessible for everyone. They include:

* asking people to ensure that they are in a private space where the group will not be overheard;

* encouraging people to feel free to turn their cameras on and off as needed, to move about or stretch or lie-down if that feels more comfortable to them;

* giving permission to look away from the screen when you need to;

* keeping to agreed beginning and end times;

* having clear agreements about joining late and leaving early and what the group has agreed is, and isn't, acceptable;

* agreeing on how you will take turns to speak;

* asking all others to mute their microphones during individual sharing.

We have included a few resources specifically about holding online spaces that are more trauma informed in the online resources section. Holding Red Tents online can also introduce barriers. Many may not have a computer, tablet, smartphone or internet available to access Red Tent meetings. How can you support or address this as a community? Others may lack the technological know-how or confidence to access an online meeting. If so, can you offer support over the phone, or find a way that a friend, carer or family member can set them up?

Technical issues can be frustrating at times, so do have a couple of practice runs using whatever online meeting platform you plan to use first. Give clear guidance at the beginning about all members muting themselves when another is speaking and what to do if the internet connection drops out. It is important to be aware that with online Red Tents, there is the chance of being overheard by others in a person's household, so encourage people to find quiet and private space if possible.

Liberation as Care

Thinking about these multiple issues that affect access to and the experience of your Red Tent is an expression of care. It also requires care to become a practice. You need to both care for one another and all those who arrive in your Red Tent space, whilst also staying aware of your own need for care as you navigate all of this.

If you recall we began with care for ourselves and each other and we did this for a reason. If we are under-resourced and unable to rest and replenish ourselves we will find navigating the change that might be triggered by this chapter difficult.

Being open to creating liberatory spaces where all are welcome in our communities requires us to challenge ourselves again and again, and we can only do that if we also know how to forgive ourselves, support ourselves, lean into support and look after our needs.

These are things that collective Red Tents can offer us and so building a culture of collective care is part and parcel of this liberation work, not separate from it or a nice-to-have extra. It is a central part of the work.

It is also a form of liberation to choose to care for ourselves as we work to create spaces that include everyone, and it's a work of liberation to make those spaces, ones where everyone can genuinely experience collective care.

REFLECTIVE QUESTIONS

★ What does creating a liberatory space mean for you? What does it mean for those you are in community with?

★ Which oppressions mentioned in this chapter do you experience?

★ Are there oppressions that you experience that we didn't concentrate on here? Do you feel left out? What would you like to say to us?

★ Which oppressions lie totally out of your own personal field of experience?

★ Are there any oppressions that lie out of the experience of your entire group?

★ Do you have any fear or anxiety about how to welcome a more diverse human experience into your group?

★ How might you make your Red Tent feel welcoming to a wider range of women in your community?

★ How will you welcome women of different ages?

★ What about women with different backgrounds? Those who are Black, Indigenous or people of colour?

★ How do you include those who speak different languages or who have different cultures or religions?

★ Have you thought about different abilities and disabilities?

★ What about those on the autistic spectrum or those living with mental health problems such as depression or anxiety?

5.

STARTING A RED TENT

At first, they weren't called Red Tents. They were just kind of new moon gatherings. It was something I started really organically with some friends. We just wanted a space where we could come together as a way to witness the new moon in our lives because, for me, that's part of what the new moon is about. It's when the skies are the darkest and so, it was an invitation to create space to look at some of the harder and more challenging parts of our lives and to share that with each other and to be there to support each other. At first, we kind of laughed about it and we would call it our "fake ritual" because it wasn't grounded in anything. It was just this thing that was spontaneous. Then when I opened Shecosystem, the women's workspace I ran in Toronto, I had this dream of it being like a Red Tent because there are just no physical places in our society where women can gather.

Emily

Emily talks about this sense she had of the desire to create a space for herself and her friends to explore whatever difficulties they may be facing in life but to do so together, in solidarity. In our experience we have also found it powerful to say things out loud in the company of others. To sit down and 'open up' is to literally reveal something hidden inside you so that you may know it more fully. If you choose to hold and initiate a Red Tent, you may recognise something similar within yourself. Perhaps you have found there is a connection you crave in your own life that you may not quite be able to describe. Maybe you long to connect with women you already know in a way that feels more honest or authentic. Perhaps you have a sense that you want to connect with women you don't know yet in this way.

Somewhere in each of us who choose to embark on this journey is a desire for a different kind of connection to other women. A sense that the way we have been taught to relate to one another isn't always giving us the types of relationships and connections with each other that we most desire.

In the families and cultures where we both grew up, the connections we had with other women earlier in our lives often involved an unspoken distance. Yes, we had female friends and family. Yes, we talked to them – sometimes a lot. But we often didn't tell them what we really knew in our hearts, what we were really feeling or what was really troubling us. Somewhere along the way we must have learnt – and many of the women around us must have learnt also – that it wasn't safe to share our full selves. In the Red Tent we invite ourselves and each other to let that go and to embrace the whole of who we are, and that means making space for myriad notions of femininity and womanhood, as multiple and complex as we all are.

We both recollect that there was competition and even rivalry. Often it wasn't spoken or expressed clearly, but we both recall a sense of not looking right and not fitting in and of comparing ourselves to others who seemed to fit in better. Again, the expectations we received from very early in our lives about what we 'should' be like or look like can be traced – via the people and messages around us – to patriarchy, to the expectations of women within it to look, behave in and be a certain way. In a world where photos can be painstakingly manipulated, social media posts can be crafted for hours to look spontaneous and celebrity culture creates an illusion of perfection, our sense of ourselves and our worth are often impacted. Resisting these judgements, whether they are received overtly or subtly from others or arising as internalised oppression within ourselves, is a seemingly small but often very challenging, and important, act of resistance.

Whether or not we actively engage with this narrative of beauty, success or popularity, it is the backdrop of many women's lives. Instead of holding our popular media, advertising industries and multinational corporations to account, we have allowed them to perpetuate feelings of inadequacy, and to cast us as enemies vying for the same limited spotlight, promotion or external validation. In the Red Tent we find that sharing more honestly helps us to drop at least some of the competition and instead find compassion and love for one another.

I welcome them in, I explain that this is a safe place where we share deeply, not in the usual way that we might talk to each other. For example, yesterday in the Red Tent a woman was saying that she always fights against women and doesn't trust them. But from coming to the Red Tent she has learnt that it is safe to be with women, that she can trust women. I believe this is because women don't know how to trust themselves, so they don't know how to begin to trust other women.

Susana

In this way, the Red Tent can support us to resist these stereotypes. But we also have to guard against others that may arise within our Tents. To make sure that we are not replacing what we learnt from our cultures with similar expectations of womanhood or femininity within our Tents. This can happen subtly, for example, when a woman provides advice over lunch around healthy eating that is rooted in a fatphobic understanding of weight and health. Or when we make assumptions about the ways that women should behave, look or feel. Lu draws our attention to how comments suggesting she might have her period or perhaps be pregnant had an impact on her, as a woman who is intersex, born with MRKH[1] and without a uterus.

The fact that anytime I would say I had a headache, or I felt sick, or I was really craving some chocolate, or, you know, by that point in my late 20s, and people would say stuff like, "Oh, pitter patter" or "Be careful!" or, you know, "Could you be...?" Like, they're just comments, but they would happen all the time and they would land like a punch in the stomach. I came up with the idea that this was a kind of reproductive closeting that's happening because we're a straight cis couple. Everyone's just asking "Why are you not having babies?" Not if or can but when.

Lu

For us, the Red Tent is also about disrupting both the do-it-all culture and also the expectations that we should be a certain way. They are a refuge for

---

1   Mayer-Rokitansky-Küster-Hauser (MRKH syndrome) affects 1 in every 4000-5000 people and is where a person is born without a uterus or with a partially formed uterus. For information and support: mrkh.org.uk

both the never-ending journey of 'to-dos' and the expectation that womanhood has one single story.

Red Tents challenge this with the invitation to come and rest, to *be*, to *do* nothing and create a space where each of us is welcome. So Red Tents aren't another workshop, much as we love and celebrate those. Our commitment to this is why we so clearly state on the Red Tent Directory website that the Tents we list respond to the wishes of those present each time they meet and are not workshops, trainings or personal development. They are about deliberately being and sharing for its own sake, and about being as honest as we choose to be in any given moment about our needs and what we want to share and offer one another.

I see the holes in society that mirror the gaps within myself; I see the cracks in community that I too grew up with. Now, I desperately want to lick and nurse these inner and outer wounds, which is why so much of my work is about belonging and creating lasting community both for my internal salve and for society's healing too. I want to feel that sense of arriving somewhere and the door swinging gladly open. I want to know that welcome mat is for me. So, when I wanted to start a Red Tent, I told myself it was all about creating a safe place for other women, a place they knew they could come to be listened to and to be loved. Of course what I realised was that I wanted this vessel for myself. I wasn't well at the time and was feeling very alone. I had had to stop doing some of the things that had, until then, kept me well-nourished. I desperately needed the Red Tent space; I needed to sit on a bean bag in someone else's house or outside on the grass surrounded by women. In time I knew deep down that if I could be vulnerable, the kindness of these women would rush in and fill me up.

I met with other folk who saw the same need in community and society for women to feel loved up and have a resting place. We set about creating a gathering that fed and nourished all those souls who were tired, fed up and over-cooked from the busy days of our lives. What we were offering struck a chord with so many people we met. A female-of-centre space in homes across the city. Although there are still holes in society and cracks in our communities, setting up a Red Tent has filled some of those fissures for me with radical loving tenderness. And I have found a calm place to return when the incline gets too steep.

Aisha

As Aisha shares, you might feel that you want to set up a Red Tent because you feel a need for nourishment and holding for yourself. You might be having a challenging time in your own life, feel isolated or just crave a place where you can show up, relax and share in the company of others.

In the few times I've attended Red Tent circles, I've come out feeling hugely energised, validated, positive, uplifted, supported, understood, valued, nurtured and loved (and moved by the ability of a couple of hours in the presence of a few other women to effect this change in me). The feeling of connection, acceptance and warmth from other women in such settings is unrivalled.
Madeleine

Whatever your reasons for starting a Red Tent, the benefits, the magic of those moments of quiet peace and resting alongside others, of being accepted as all of who you are, are in our experience, worth the time and commitment necessary to start a Red Tent.

I've received so much from doing this, way more than I ever expected.
Lou

We believe that these spaces where women can connect honestly and take time and space for themselves are critically important in our cultures at this time. They are not just radical because they are unusual for some of us, but because they help us to restore and recharge ourselves. We have also found that they help us to show up for the rest of our lives in a different way.

I was introduced to the Red Tent a few months after the birth of my son. I needed to talk, I needed to be around other mothers to share experiences and learn from one another. That's when I discovered the meaning of Sisterhood.
Pascale

A sense of shared sisterhood is apparent in many Red Tent spaces as women come together to connect and support one another. The underlying fuel for this sisterly relationship is a loving acceptance of each other, even though there maybe challenges and lessons to learn together around the corner.

I've learned that by putting my simple and core need – to be held and respected by a group of like-minded women – as prime place on my calendar, I am better able to thrive and grow in other areas of my life. It puts peace at the centre for me.
Ali

What might inspire you to create or join a Red Tent in your community? Only you know. But chances are you might have felt, in your own life, the pain of that which you have left unspoken. Or the exhaustion of trying to do it all. Chances are you might crave an honest space to *be* rather than to *do*. A space where existing is enough. A space where things can arise in the moment. A space that nourishes and supports you. A space, most simply, where women are invited to meet.

We think of many of us doing this, across the globe, as a simple practice of creating small ripples that can support more widespread change. Something which, through drawing on many practices that women have held together in the past, helps us to find a different way to be with and support one another. A way to share and connect.

To help you map out your own needs if you want to be part of creating a Red Tent yourself, one of the questions that we invite you to ask is about what is personally motivating you to do this at this time? Asking this can be helpful in getting clarity for yourself.

Preparing yourself to find your Sisters

Some questions you might want to reflect on as you begin to call your Tent into being:

★ What are your personal motivations for wanting to be an initiator of a Red Tent?

★ What do you think a Red Tent would bring to your life?

★ Why now? Why here?

★ How do you think the Red Tent you are envisioning might be situated within a community you are part of?

★ How might your Red Tent be collectively held?

★ How can you invite cooperation, support and solidarity as you bring it into being?

★ What, if anything, do you feel that you are reclaiming or remembering? From where and from whom?

Building a Collective Vision

We want to encourage you to think about creating a collectively held Red Tent space as a way to disrupt the sense many of us have that to get something done we have to go it alone. By doing it together we are refusing to participate in the paradigm that we need to expend ourselves to make something happen. Instead we think of intentionally calling in our sisters and committing to growing something together.

I've been running a Red Tent almost every month. Every time a new woman has offered her house, garden or place under an olive tree for the occasion.

Susan

We invite you to think deliberately about collectively held Tents that a group of women run and look after together because we have learnt, over time, that it is the Red Tents which are run by a group of women that seem to have longevity. It is also these that can catch us, as holders of space, when we ourselves need to be held and supported. They don't rely on us to be constantly full of energy and taking the lead. Instead collectively held spaces allow us to take a back seat when we need to, to rest and recover and be part of a team.

I began to resent being the one to hold the Red Tent alone when I had nowhere to go. I loved seeing women value the space I had created, but I wished that I had that too. My role in the Tent had been, from the beginning, that of a facilitator – the holder of the space. So when times arose that I wanted the space to be held for me, this was not available. I couldn't have a bad day because I was expected to be the one that was on it.
Su

As you begin to think about crafting your own Red Tent, we invite you think about doing the groundwork first and to consider calling in one or two people who you think might be able to hold the vision for starting a Red Tent with you. If you already run a Red Tent and feel like you are doing it solo you can always make a decision to invite in one or two new people who you think might be able to hold a shared vision with you, even if you have been 'going it alone' for years.

We realised it was going to be really hard work for just the two of us. And so, we looked around the people who came to the circle and picked a few and [invited them to join us to create] a little mini support circle within the larger circle to help support the Red Tent. We'd hold confidentiality and it would be done with the same kind of level of respect as the wider Red Tent, so we could build trust and hold the sort of container that we wanted it to be.
Laura

We recommend that you start by getting together to think about what your shared vision for the Red Tent might be. We also suggest that you start with the big picture of what you are hoping to create, before diving into the details and practicalities. Here are some things to think about when inviting other women to hold a Red Tent with you:

✳ it helps to talk through what skills you have and what skills they have – to see if your skills and the things that you are passionate about complement each other;

✳ it helps if you share a similar intent in co-creating the Tent and if you can share honestly with one another what you hope to get out of co-creating this and what you are hoping to build. You might also think of building slowly with a small group in the beginning;

✳ it helps if you share with them your values and motivation…and perhaps also this book or other resources about Red Tents. See our list of resources at the end of the book.

It can take time to find the right sisters and to make this happen. It can also take some processing of our own fear about what might happen if we really do this, if we really create space and invite women to join us. In our experience, you may hear all sorts of voices in your head like *What if no one comes?* or *What if they don't understand or want to join me?*

We believe that collectively held Red Tents work well because they are self-evolving, based on shared ownership and collective involvement. For this reason it is worth spending a bit of time thinking about how you can build a solid foundation for your Tent, as well as thinking about more practical elements like where you will hold your Tents, how you will run them and how you plan to tell other women about them and invite them to come?

However, you might feel inspired to get started and find that you don't come across the right people to organise a Tent collectively with at the outset. If this happens, we suggest you start a Tent anyway, however small it may be to begin with, but continue to hold the vision of birthing a collectively held Red Tent. If you commit to holding Red Tents and inviting women for a period of time, which we will discuss in more detail in the pages that follow, some women will likely show up who are willing and able to hold the vision with you.

Don't try to do it all. Please don't try to do it all. This plea comes from years of working with, seeing, observing and being a woman who has tried to do it all. I can honestly say that it makes us less effective, as well as exhausting us and wearing us out. It's a lose-lose situation.

Mary Ann

Creating a Shared Intention

When you are thinking about the group of women who hold and organise your Red Tent, we want to invite you to think about developing some principles of collective community leadership to help orientate the organising of a Tent collectively amongst a group of women.

We have learnt that it's important that whatever holding structure you have and however you name it, you think about how to intentionally and deliberately support one another in the kind of collective leadership which allows you all to not only lead but also to be nourished and resourced by the experience of being part of a Red Tent.

We hold it to be the case that all of us want and need to feel held, heard and seen. When we don't feel this we can lurch from feeling undervalued and like *everyone is getting nourished and supported by this Red Tent thing apart from me* to the thought that *I (alone) need to make sure everyone else gets what they need from this.*

These are ways that women, probably for generations, have responded to the expectation in our cultures that women would do most, if not all, of the caring work. Much of what women, and especially women of colour, have done from overseeing the natural processes of welcoming new life as midwives, to caring for others in death, providing healing medicine for the sick to cooking daily food for family and community, is valuable care work to be uplifted. But this desire in us to care can get out of balance. We still find many women employed in the caring professions and domestic activities which are often not only poorly paid but may be in contractual arrangements that are unstable and inequitable. Meanwhile in a family it is often assumed that a female member will care for unwell relatives, reduce her hours to look after a growing child and get the dinner on the table, whether she works full time or not.

For many women caring for others is a fulfilling part of their life. We may feel loved and needed in this way. Many of us feel we have a strong bond of empathy with our families, community and often with the natural world. But however fulfilling, this role in society can at times be thankless and restrictive. It may also limit our creativity, stifle our freedom and restrict our possibilities. Moreover, these social and cultural realities have contributed to an experience that we and many other women we know have had of finding that we resort to being a carer almost as default and that this has become an unhealthy pattern. It can lead to us styling ourselves as rescuers, even in situations where we are experiencing abuse or victimisation.

For many years being the carer and one to sort everything out for others was a very dominant narrative in my life, and became, in many ways, the only way in which I felt my life had value. This belief led me into situations which I now recognise were abusive and caused me harm. They also became harmful and toxic for the other people in them. I now know that when I could only see myself as carer and fixer I was denying a part of myself that needed to be cared for and that in doing so I was also performing a very real feminine conditioning to be a caretaker who neglected her own needs.

Mary Ann

Many women who create Red Tents have many years of skills and experiences that they can bring around facilitating spaces for women to meet. They can find themselves stepping into a space of leading and holding and creating alone because of this.

I realise now the mistake I had made. What I had done was create a free workshop rather than a Red Tent. I had created a space where women expected to show up and that I would have it all planned for them. They were structured, themed, and resourced. And I always knew my stuff. I was significantly out of pocket having paid for venues and materials, books, films, craft supplies. I made soup, provided tea and massaged hands – and only ever accepted donations in return – which rarely covered the costs. I had not created a communal shared space, where women felt empowered to step forward and contribute, but I had very successfully created a safe and held space, facilitated by me. I had invested huge amounts of my time, energy and money for nearly 20 years in gathering what I knew. Now I was devaluing myself. Giving away what I had to offer, not only for free, but at cost to myself. I had been a strong advocate of women acknowledging their own worth – and here I was devaluing mine.

Su

We want to invite you to deliberately turn this expectation on its head and create a space where women can care for themselves…together. This, as we have said, is radical work. A world that accommodates a wider number of ways of being a woman is one in which we can support each other to live beyond these stereotypes.

We can, in the Red Tent, create a space outside those realms which is creative, expansive and nurturing. We are challenging our conditioning. And those of us who hold and organise Red Tents can also easily find ourselves slipping back into habitual, learnt ways of being if we don't put safeguards in place to prevent this from happening.

It is a place where ego, professional 'hats' and baggage are left at the front door with all the demands of life. The women's space offers a monthly sacred and safe space where you can reconnect with your inner self, the divine feminine within you and connect with other like-minded women. This space allows us to deeply exhale and breathe in much needed prana to carry us through until the next new moon.

Sanita

We see these patterns show up in Red Tents. Even though we want to resist them. It's radical work, challenging our own conditioning and ultimately that of the culture around us. Our conditioning may have us either trying to do everything to make sure everyone else gets what they need or feeling resentful about everyone else getting what they need when we feel that we are not.

We can't necessarily stop this coming up as an issue, but we can anticipate it and hold one another intentionally in it as a collective leadership group. We can also take action around it. Doing this collectively is the first action. By holding Red Tents collectively, we lessen any leaders' sense of being a lone martyr for a cause, caretaking everyone else or holding it all.

Calling the Circle

For me, equality is essential. The circle is the perfect form in that it is already equal and invites nothing more of us as sisters than to see and be seen; to listen and be heard; to share equally.

Lu

We use the term circle to describe a gathering or Red Tent and to reflect a sense of flattening the hierarchy of the space. It denotes the way of sitting together in a circle formation. It feels also like a natural way to come together when there are more than a few people. You can see everyone's faces and it suggests a certain flow of conversation with everyone having equal part in it. We are not saying that hierarchy does not exist in relation to knowledge, privilege, experience or age but that the way of sitting together in the round means there is not a speaker and an audience. Each woman takes her turn to speak, each woman has access to being heard, each woman can listen to the person speaking without interrupting them. It is a way of democratising the space and allowing inclusive involvement. In this way it forms more than a gathering of voices round the fire or kitchen table. It also draws on many indigenous traditions that sit in and have sat in this way to hold counsel. [2]

We always let people know that this is a specific circle for this day: it's a co-created container. There's a beginning and end. And that you can take care of your needs. We were really clear on this: it's not like the space is so sacred that you have to be scared to be yourself. I have been to women's circles where there's this feeling that we all have to act a certain way, and I have to pee but I really shouldn't get up because I'm going to be breaking the circle. Here we are like, "Go pee, go get more food!" It was really about ease and self-care, about nurturing ourselves and each other.

Emily

Bringing the practice of sitting in circle for sharing our collective vision

---

2   We would like to extend our thanks to *Calling the Circle,* Christina Baldwin, thecircleway.net for ideas on circle form, process and lineage.

is a resilient way of building community. Within the format of meeting in this simple way you can slow down the pace, invite some quiet to listen to what is present, and create the threads of connection. In short it is powerful and flexible to the needs of the group and the moments as they arise. To prevent the sense of *doing it all* and *no one supporting me* from emerging in the group, it's often helpful to create a holding circle in which we can intentionally name and hold this risk and communicate about it. In this holding circle we as organisers and holders of Tents get to be heard, seen and held. We get to explore these patterns in ourselves, and we get to consciously reject them as we hold space and responsibility collectively. We get to admit them. Laugh about them. Care for the parts of ourselves that feel like we want to rescue everyone else or feel fed up and unappreciated and in doing so hold space for change, for doing things differently.

A holding circle is a space in which any woman who may feel there is too much being expected of her by others or herself, can name it and have that heard and seen by the group. It is also a space in which we can name and share our instincts to care for everyone else first, to make sure everyone else is alright and, consciously or unconsciously, to forget about ourselves.

Red Tent St Albans hold gatherings of their 'Guardians Circle' which they call 'camp fires'. Meanwhile in the Brighton Red Tent the 'Steering Circle', as it was called, arose out of a need to share the work of creating the Red Tent, without it feeling like a fully administrative or practical thing. As Aisha explains,

We almost got to the stage where the core group of us that set up the Brighton Red Tent reached peak email capacity and we realised that taking our discussions offline into an intentionally held space would not only nurture ourselves but provide a place where we could discuss ideas together. We were able to plan for future Red Tents and embed a sense of collective ownership for the community. We did so by training up people so they could share the holding and hosting of each gathering. We called it the 'steering circle' because we had a clear sense of our collective vision and our responsibility as those who were organising the Red Tent but without a hierarchy of being the centre of it. The centre was always the Red Tent community and we were gently steering the ship along on calm waters, or, at times, on turbulent seas.

Making a Commitment

We created the first Red Tent event at my house. It was really good...but then it took some time to establish. In fact, it kind of flopped for about a year after that. We'd have a Red Tent and maybe two or three women would show up or only one woman would come. And it didn't feel like it was running. It felt a bit uncomfortable. Personally, it also took me a long time to normalise the word Red Tent in my family and my community and start to talk to people about it myself.

I spoke to Aisha and asked, "What do I need to do?" She said, just commit to six Red Tents. Put six Red Tents in the diary. You must both be at all six Red Tents, whether anyone else is there or not. If you commit to them, the women will come. And that's what happened. The women started coming. We'd host them in different women's houses and one of us would gently hold the space. From there it established itself. We started creating a mailing list and it grew pretty quickly. We've now got about 300 women on it!

Mads

Just like a newly turned allotment, your first few Red Tents will be about sowing seeds, weeding and watering. Watching the flourishing of your Red Tent will take commitment, inspiration and time.

My life both at work and home is full of wonderful men but scarce few women. I knew nothing about Red Tents and I was anxious about going, wondering what the other women would make of me, but so pleasantly surprised at the genuine gentle welcome and acceptance of me just as I am. I never dreamed I'd create a group myself! ... At the start of last year, I summoned up the courage and invited three friends over, talked to them about my idea and started from there. In 18 months we have grown from a group of four women to about 15, and there are usually about eight in our circle at any one time, depending on who's doing what on the dates we meet.

Lara

As with the seasons, your efforts will pass through cycles of their own: welcoming women; noticing those who stay or just visit once; experiencing disappointment if things don't meet your expectations; and bathing in joy at the simplicity of sharing and being with other women. All the while you are holding the intention to provide a space for women to turn up, as they are, and for you to turn up, just as you are too.

It can take time for roots to grow, for consistency and momentum to take hold, so be kind and patient with yourself and others. It may be a while before you begin to taste the fruits of your offerings. So, keep this in your intentions as you follow this path of bringing a Red Tent to the women of your community.

What I have to keep doing is holding the space. That's really what I have to offer at the moment, is holding them and hopefully, like you say, three committed people will emerge and maybe they'll all come one time together, which would be really good!

So often it's just me and another woman, sometimes me and two women. One Red Tent, six women barrelled through the door: I had no idea they were coming! Someone had brought someone who brought someone who brought someone. That was really nice to have more people in the space. And one time nobody came, so I held the Red Tent with my husband, which was really lovely, although a little unconventional!

Susannah

Over the years of supporting women to create Red Tent spaces in their communities we have learnt that it helps to start with a commitment to holding a Red Tent and inviting women to it for a specific period of time. This feels important to us because Red Tents do vary in how quickly they thrive. Some women find it takes time for their Tent to grow and put down roots. Others find that they grow very quickly.

I remember at the beginning that we said to each other: We'll give it a year, we'll commit to a year…and if it doesn't work, we'll drop it. We really didn't know whether there was just going to be me and Laura sat there with one or two other people. In fact, it was like a little spark and then it just grew.

Lou

You might want to commit for a year initially. You might find six months more manageable. That's okay too. What is important is that you commit to holding your Tent for a period of time and opening it to women in your community, those you know, and perhaps also those you don't know yet. So, figure out what your commitment to your Tent is at the outset: is it six months, twelve months or perhaps thirteen moon cycles which is just a bit longer than a calendar year?

Offering the Invitation

There were months when no woman showed up, so I meditated on my own and focused on myself; sometimes it was easy to accept it, sometimes I didn't like it and resisted it.

There were months when one woman showed up, so it was a one-to-one rather than a circle and interesting conversations happened, revealing unexpected coincidences in our lives that just blew me away.

There were months when two women came, so it was a triangle rather than a circle, but it started having the feeling of a community and it was pleasant and encouraging.

There were months when three women came, so it was a square and it felt more stable and grounded than the triangle, but still very magical.

There were months when four women showed up and it started being a real circle and I felt successful, but also more challenged in running it.

There were months when five women came and I felt super exuberant, as it felt like I had a full house!

Gabriella

One of the things that can inspire fear in us is making the invitation to other women to join us. It isn't surprising. The idea of calling other women to do something that, as we have explored, is – on some level – is a radical act is likely to challenge you in one way or another. Know that it is normal to feel some resistance about this. Even if you are the kind of person who is used to inviting women to the workshops that you run, or to parties you hold, inviting them into a Red Tent space may still feel different and difficult.

We have found that it helps before you start to get clear for yourself about what it is you want to create and why. Hopefully reading this book will help you with this, but we also recommend you start by doing your own thinking and reflection about it too. Even if you don't have anyone to share it with at the outset, it's helpful to write about it or reflect on it as a means of getting clear for yourself.

REFLECTIVE QUESTIONS

✷ What do you want your Red Tent to feel like?

✷ What do you hope that the Red Tent will create in your life and the lives of other women?

✷ What do you want the 'culture' of your Red Tent to be like? How is this similar or different to what you observe and experience in other parts of your life?

✷ What traditions, learning and experience are you bringing to your Red Tent space?

✷ What traditions, learning and experience do you need to honour, in your Red Tent space?

6.

BRINGING YOUR IDEAS TO LIFE

Women looking to start a Red Tent often have many practical questions. Those who already run them may now be wondering how the approach we are proposing impacts the practicalities and practices of running a Red Tent. In this section we take a look at those.

Choosing a Space

The first question is usually: *Where should we hold it?*

We have heard of Red Tents happening in homes, community spaces, on the land and in venues offered by women who own or manage them for other purposes and – as you'll read below – in various outside spaces as well. We envision Red Tents happening in schools and universities, in prisons and refugee camps. With a little creativity, anywhere that women meet a Red Tent can be born.

In identifying a location for an in-person Red Tent, we invite you to think about a safe and nurturing space which can hold the circle of women that you want to bring together. It doesn't necessarily have to be an ideal space, but a space where a number of women can sit physically in a circle together is important.

It's great to be in a space where you can share and be supported by other women in total confidence without any agenda. To top it all I have met some really inspiring women.

Renée

You want to think too about how you might make it comfortable, either by using the furniture and resources that are already in the space or by inviting women to bring their own cushions or pop up chairs to sit on. Once your Red Tent becomes established, you might collect or purchase a collection of things which could include materials for decorating, as well as seating equipment and so forth.

Red Tent Physical Spaces.
Things to Consider:

Whether or not you can find a space that meets all your ideal requirements, it is important to be aware of the choices you are making, particularly if you plan to host your Tent each month in a publicly hired space that has a regular cost.

* **Geographical accessibility:** How will people get there? Is it close to public transport or will they need to drive? Is there free and accessible parking available?

* **Finances:** What are the costs and how will they be covered on an on-going basis?

* **Physical Accessibility:** When identifying a space, it's important to think about accessibility issues. When looking for a space consider who would be able to physically access the space and who might not. Does it have stairs? If so, is there a lift or ramp for those with mobility issues?

* **Decorations:** Some Red Tents are ornately decorated, others use very simple decorations or props. This is also something to think about when identifying a space and is something we will cover in more detail in the next chapter.

At Home

Many Red Tents take place in women's homes, often rotating hosts around the group month to month. This is a sustainable way of creating shared connections and community, and also sharing responsibility for hosting each month. We have seen many Tents start in homes and there is a simplicity to this. For example, it can be as simple as just make some space to sit down, put a sign on the door saying welcome, and put the kettle on! Also, after the Red Tent is finished and everything is packed away, many women share how wonderful it feels that it took place in their home at all. Almost as if there is a sense of "wow did that really happen in this room?" as they look around at the lounge that housed a circle of women rearranged back to its daily functionality.

Caversham Red Tent has moved venues and locations to adapt to the needs of the community and as attendance increased.

Practically speaking, we started in a venue that I use for yoga classes but it wasn't cosy enough. We moved to my lounge where we were for the next three years until we outgrew it. Then we tried the yurt over a summer and because it's such a magical space, everyone opted to stay on through last winter, despite needing to use a compost toilet (not to everyone's liking!) and needing private transport to get there. The women bring cushions, blankets, treats to share. I dream one day of having a dedicated place where the sanctity of the space is built up over time and the energy is not interrupted by lots of other activities. However, the yurt is mainly used in the day by teenage boys who have been excluded from school and I only feel that on some level this adds to the special nature of the space.
Tessa

Inviting women into our homes doesn't work for everyone or every community. For some, the idea of inviting other women, particularly those they may not have met, into their home doesn't feel positive and nurturing. You may feel weighed down by the idea of organising the arrangements with those you share your home with, or worried about being disturbed by them. Sorting the house out for visitors can feel too much. You may feel that there will be too much to do to decorate the house if you host it at your home. You may feel your house isn't suitable either in size or location. Not all women live in a place that is easy for others to get to, and parking and public transport can be challenging. Many women also feel unsafe sharing their address with those they don't yet know. And meeting in women's homes can add to the sense that a Red Tent is for a specific type of woman, with a specific class background, racial identity or level of privilege.

When it's at someone's house, it could be maybe a barrier ... especially if you're going to someone's house and there's lots of people that know each other and have been to that house before and you've never been there. If you go to a community centre, it's a neutral place which I think works quite well.

I think it can become a thing if you're hosting and it has to be a certain way and maybe if your house isn't as nice as someone else's house, you can start to feel like you don't want to host because there's just a lot of pressure, for example when and where does your family go? We had it at one woman's house and her kids were all up in the bedroom upstairs trying to keep out the way while the husband or partner had to go out. It's lovely to do from time to time, but when that's always the expectation, I think it can be a bit much – especially because we were doing it in the evening for two and a half hours – to fit in with people's lives.

Lily

These worries are common. Knowing that we are not alone in our fears helps. At the end of the day to host a Red Tent in your home it doesn't need to be tidy, spotless, large or decorated. Rather the Red Tent is all about *being* and not *doing* so to allow your home to be just the way it is can in itself be liberating! To support women to host at home some Red Tents have also found ways to address issues by creating a culture of collective support with setting up the space, putting it back to normal and helping with childcare. Some also establish practices for address sharing which avoid personal addresses being shared in public invitations but instead send them by text only to those women who have signed up to attend.

Many of us feel scared of meeting new people: the pause before you enter a room, the numbers that never get dialled. It is a big deal trying something new particularly in a society which values individual thinking and in which even our self-help books tell us that only you have the power to change your life. But we can also think of ourselves as part of a web that spans through our history and interweaves with one another's lives. Didn't we evolve in community? Didn't we grow through passing on what we'd learnt? Didn't our shared stories create our collective identity?

That is why we believe that the feeling of coming home that you can experience through going to a Red Tent, by dialling that number and knocking on that door is a powerful act. It is an act of rebellion from the rhetoric of isolation. It is looking head-on at loneliness, addressing the hunger for connection and trusting that a stranger can love you. By stepping through that door, by entering a Red Tent, you honour our collective history of being women in the world and all those that walked this earth before us.

For those who are able, inviting women into our homes can be a way to challenge the ways in which our culture separates us. It is a little like the moment you invite a new friend through the door: it marks a stage in your friendship, indicates a willingness to commit to them being in your life for a while to come. With Red Tents the preamble is shorter perhaps, an email exchange or phone call and then a new person you haven't met before is welcomed through your door. What is more startling is that after spending time in circle, the sizzle and crackle of connection is made and that stranger leaves as a friend. This, quite simply, is how community is born. It is a mix of shyness, courage and a bold act to light the fuse of exchange. And through the recent Covid-19 global pandemic, we have learnt that this can happen online too!

Pets

Be aware if hosting at home that different people have strong feelings and needs about pets – some women may have allergies to pet hair, others may have anxiety around certain animals. Be sure that pets are not in the space you are using for Red Tent, including the entrance hall or front yard, until you are sure that they will not be an issue for any of the women attending.

Public Spaces

If for any reason inviting women into your home doesn't feel like the most resonant way to organise your Red Tent, or if it has outgrown a home setting, it's important to find an alternative space that will allow you to have an experience of ease for yourself in the organisation of your Tent.

Some Tents do decide that a shared public space is preferable and meets their needs much better. If you are choosing to rent a space, you need to think about costs. This may affect the length of your Tent and the way that you organise it: how will the community fund the space and make sure that meeting in this way is sustainable?

You can collect donations from women attending your Tent to cover the costs of a venue, like the Paris Red Tent does, running a number of Tents across the city that meet at civic centres.

We just have to pay five pounds an hour, so I used to just put a cup out for a few coins each. I'd always say bring a blanket and a cushion and your favourite tea bag and then people would just bring their own stuff and what they needed. Usually it was one or two pounds in the pot. And then if we had extra money left over, I'd roll it over for when people forget or if there's one time it doesn't cover the cost. I found it worked really well in the community hall, for me. Also it was good having it on the community centre timetable as a women's circle happening that night if new people wanted to come. I felt like it made it feel more accessible.
Lily

Perhaps someone in your network has access to a space that you can use for free or on a donation basis. Another Tent we spoke with meets at a yoga studio that is run by one of its founders. Some Red Tents find that, over time, their needs, in terms of the space where they meet, change as well. If you do make changes to your venue, remember to consult regular attenders. City-centre based venues may work better for people if transport links are good. However, finding affordable and accessible venues can present challenges for organisers too.

The Red Tent started off at Swansea University when the original organisers were students there. When they graduated, they no longer had the free use of the room, so it moved to a small therapy centre in central Swansea. This is where it lived for a few years until the business was sold, and again the venue was no longer available. From then, it moved to people's homes, while we looked for a new central venue.

Michelle

Outside Tents

That morning, the fire in the garden was, for me, just about the best welcome I could imagine. Fire in the morning seems somehow more powerful than it does at night. The women were a diverse and gorgeous bunch: from young women beginning their careers to women recently become mothers, to those traversing menopause and embracing their elder energy. We were invited to call in our ancestors: living, dead, biologically and spiritually connected to us. I lit a candle bringing in my grandmothers, my mother, my sisters, my friends. It was a beautiful sharing of who we are in our lineage and so profound to acknowledge those who have come before us. The ancient past and the budding future was held so powerfully and lightly in the glory and tangle of the present that it was all welcomed. This holding, this experiencing so many parallel and complementary stories with love and respect, is for me what it means to create sacred space.

Steph

Many Red Tents are hosted outside during the warmer months and there is something powerful about really getting away from the usual dramas of everyday life by stepping outside. Often our desire to get in touch with ourselves and each other can extend to finding some connection with nature. When Tents happen outside they often don't need decorating as they are already dressed in the colours of nature! As Susan shares with us, being outside can make it feel very simple and effective to create an inviting place to be.

I bought a whole load of little red Turkish carpets that you can sit on. I used some beautiful red material and wrapped it between four or five trees which helped to make a Red Tent shape. And that's where I had my first Red Tent.

Susan

Weather is always going to be a factor here, but if you are able to find somewhere with a shelter nearby, then having a fire outside or meeting in a pretty spot can be a lovely way to gather. When I, Aisha, was in Brighton we held a number of Red Tents outside in the summer months which was a rich experience in many ways. It was glorious to be immersed in nature, and there was enough space to spread out. Often there was a waiting list to attend Red Tents as the community grew quite quickly, but when they were held outside each gathering could accommodate a large gathering of women. As well as room to have a big group of people, there was real beauty in having the birds and wind providing a backdrop to our quiet time together. The enjoyment of being outside extended into a weekday Red Tent that included a walk. This gave scope for smaller group sharing as well as reflection time afterwards.

Brighton Red Tent was also fortunate to have the Brighton Red Yurt, which was created by Jill, a driving force of the Red Tent community and financed in part by collective fundraising. This provided a place for women to go for quiet during their monthly bleed, as well as workshop space, forty minutes outside of the city. Numerous Red Tents were held there in the summer, and the location provided an element of freedom to the gatherings as well as the pleasure of being outside at such an abundant time of year. When meeting in this way we felt connected to women from the past, our ancestors, who might have met together in nature to honour the passing seasons, significant life transitions and to share wisdom and stories. We felt connected to them and honoured their practices with our own.

It may be that finding time to be outside at night brings a special quality to your Red Tent too. As Lara explains in describing her Red Tent in Cilgerran, Wales.

Being together in circle around a fire is really special... The flames can make the whole circle feel different than it might by candlelight or under the sun. The mood is different – slower – as the fire somehow gives a space for us to sink down a little more deeply on the inside and as a group. We are reminded that spaces of silence are fine, with just the crackling of the logs and each woman contemplating the embers, switching off from everyday concerns or quietly feeling a little deeper into what she doesn't give space to in the hurry of everyday life, knowing that she can voice it when she is ready…there is time.

Lara

Red Tents Online

When I first dreamed of an online Red Tent it was 2015 and I had just given birth. I'd also recently moved and didn't feel ready to create or join one out of the house. I wanted the Tent to come to me! By that stage I'd already spent years doing deep work online so I knew what was possible. But at the time I found it hard to convince others to join me virtually. Wind forward to this moment of a global pandemic and I'm so grateful we have the technology that makes connecting deeply at this time possible.

Mary Ann

During the Covid-19 pandemic, in the midst of which we are writing, many Red Tents, at least for the time being, have shifted online. Women have been innovating using the available technology and figuring out how to create an online space that feels as safe and nurturing as possible. We have seen many Tents create beautiful online offerings that have enabled women to continue to meet in the context of the pandemic.

For us at the Red Tent Directory, Red Tents are about creating spaces to be together and if we take this way of connecting online we need to do it with intention and in the same spirit in which we would meet in person. And so later in the book we will include some tips for translating what you might do in person into an online space.

We held the Red Tent online, still with some hesitation on whether or not it was going to be the same – would it feel unnatural? As we opened the space, we saw some familiar faces but also new women who had responded to the calling from far away, those who had planned on numerous past occasions to join us, but distance or schedules made it impossible, and now they were 'here'. We started our meeting, and technicalities were no longer an issue, everything flowed just as naturally and deep and healing as it usually is. As we were closing this first online attempt, all the women were thankful for this space. We were already considering gathering more frequently. It made us feel so great that this experiment was actually transforming into a new reality. It seems that as long as there is a woman with an open heart, in the same space or far apart, the red ribbons of the Red Tent will always work their magic around.

Katrina, Sophie and Bera

Tents Within Institutional Settings

Anywhere where women meet a regular space where we can share and connect without being *fixed* or critiqued can be created. We envisage Tents meeting in workplaces, schools, places of worship, community halls and marketplaces.

One of our hopes for Red Tents is that they could provide group spaces in contexts where women have been separated from their home or family and the need for safety and sisterhood are at an all-time high. For example, in places such as care homes, refugee camps, prisons, young offenders centres and detention centres where privacy and quiet may be hard to come by and connections may be strained. Perhaps Red Tents might help to counter some of the loneliness and isolation that can dramatically impact mental health and wellbeing.

We believe Red Tents could potentially be a format that could help create a space that women collectively contribute to, fostering a sense of belonging and community. We hope that sharing the simple format of meeting in this way and the opportunity for judgement-free space to speak will encourage many to start Red Tents in diverse settings.

REFLECTIVE QUESTIONS

★ How do you personally feel about hosting your Red Tent in your home?

★ If you'd prefer a communal space how might you identify one? Are there spaces in your community that you think would work well?

★ Is there a Red Tent you would like to help create in an institutional context?

★ How do you feel about meeting online to create these kinds of connection?

★ What things do you want to bear in mind when identifying space?

Identifying a Schedule

The next question is usually: *When should we hold our Red Tent and how long should it be?* The length and timing of your gatherings is an important practicality to consider as you prepare to start your Tent.

The length of Red Tent events can vary, with some lasting all or most of a day, and others being shorter and lasting for two to three hours. Some happen in the evenings, others during the day or at a weekend. What is important, when making your initial commitment, is to make an agreement about this – you can always agree to review and continue to adjust as you go. Each Red Tent usually has a beginning and end – as we will discuss in more details later in the book and most Tents invite those attending to make sure that they can stay for the duration of the time.

Moon Guided

Many Red Tents time their meetings in relation to the cycles of the moon, reflecting the ancient connections human beings have made between moon cycles and the many different cycles of our lives. This gives a regularity and a reminder that we are a part of nature and her cycles.

Some groups hold the event on the day of the new moon, others on the full moon. And others on the same day of the week each month choosing the date on that day that falls nearest to the new or full moon. Others ignore the moon cycles entirely and simply choose the first Saturday of each month, or the second Wednesday. There are no hard and fast rules about this but part of making a commitment to holding your Red Tent for a period of time is making an agreement about how you will decide when it will happen and ideally, sketching out dates for that period of time so that you can all put them in your diaries.

The earliest peoples understood that the power of life lay in the darkness of the moon... The moon with its repeating cycles of waxing and waning, became a symbol to the ancients for the birth, growth, death and renewal of all life forms... The moon, in her transformations, mirrors the same fluctuations of increase and decrease that take place in the human body and in the psyche.
Demetra George [1]

Holding a Red Tent gathering at the dark moon just before the new moon – or around that time – can, as Emily says, "create space to look at some of the harder and more challenging parts of our lives and to share that with each other and to be there to support each other."

Demetra George also points out, "We have been taught to fear and resist the decreasing energies represented by the dark, by decay, birth and death, and the unconscious. Thus, we have lost our knowledge of an essential part of the cyclical life processes, symbolised by the dark phase of the moon." [2]

---

1   George, Demetra. *Mysteries of the Dark Moon: The Healing Power of the Dark Goddess*
2   As above.

Using the lunar cycle to guide the timing for women's gatherings also honours the sense of resonance that many women feel in the cycles of the moon that seem to mirror those in our own bodies. As the moon performs her cycles, we cycle ourselves as our hormones fluctuate in their own rhythms of waxing and waning.

But, let's be clear: the cycle of the moon is predictable and menstrual cycles when we have them, vary. Meanwhile, research suggests that it's not the case that our cycles follow the moon in a predictable way or that women's cycles always synchronise. [3]

While we can see some similarities between our menstrual cycles to the moon, for us this connection is about resonance, about us connecting to something in nature that cycles in a way that is familiar to us in our own bodies. It is not an exact mirror, but a shared kind of experience, you could say.

So whilst holding Red Tents on a moon cycle also honours the menstrual cycle, which is often similar in length to that of the moon, it is important to bear in mind that not all women who attend your Red Tent will experience a menstrual cycle or be bleeding, and that even those who are will have cycles of varying lengths.

By contrast moon cycles can also be tracked by anyone, whether they menstruate or not. As a trans woman, Persia shares her reflections on the way in which some cis women's focus on the moon as forming a deep part of their connection to womanhood.

The thing is that connection to the moon cycle maybe something. But if that is used as a way to identify some group of people as being more worthy than others, because of this unproven but sensed connection with lunar cycles, then we have a problem. When it's being used as some sort of sense of belonging into the greater cosmos, I totally agree with that. But to say that it's matched within a body and that it makes those people more worthy of womanliness than others, that's a problem.

Persia

3   Hill, Maisie. *Period Power: Harness Your Hormones and Get Your Cycle Working for You*

Some writers[4] associate our bleeding time with the dark moon, linking the experience many women have of menstruation as a time to become quieter, to rest, to look after themselves and to reflect with this part of the cycle of the moon. This doesn't mean that we 'should' all be menstruating at the new moon or that this has to be when we hold our Red Tents.

Reds Tent are also sometimes held on the full moon. This time has been associated more with ovulation in women's cycles, a more outward energy a time when they feel more inclined to connect with others, whereas during menstruation they feel more inward looking. This makes sense if we consider that before artificial light, there was much more vision on full moon nights.

Remember also that many women experience pain or complications, emotional and physical associated with their menstrual cycles for a variety of different reasons and may not wish to honour their cycles in the same way.

We can hold this relationship loosely and take what is useful from it without making assumptions about the importance of when, how and whether we bleed in determining the timing of Red Tents. Assuming someone else has the same experience as you can very quickly become a barrier and cause of confusion between us. There are many ways to experience both womanhood and menstruation.

For us, when women align with an undisputed natural cycle of the moon orbiting the earth, perhaps we are asserting that women's cycles and other physical transitions that mark our lives should become part of our common language and socially accepted conversation.

REFLECTIVE QUESTIONS

✦ How will you decide when your Red Tent is held?

✦ What traditions or practices are you inspired by in this?

✦ How will you come to an agreement with your co-holders about this?

---

4   See for example Pope, Alexandra and Wurlitzer, Sjanie Hugo. *Wild Power: Discover the Magic of Your Menstrual Cycle and Awaken the Feminine Path to Power*

Sharing About Your Red Tent

Within a month we had many women on our email list and our first Red Tent was attended by twenty-two women. It took many months before each one of us holding the space each month could step back and feel nourished by a Red Tent held by others.

Aisha

It is worth thinking through at the outset how you will communicate with other women about your Red Tent. Essentially when it comes to letting people know about your Red Tent, we would like to invite you to go big and tell everyone! Red Tents are about laying out a welcome mat to women in your community so that they feel able to come whether they know someone else who is attending or not. But first you need to consider what are the breadcrumbs that you will put out there to entice people, to help people to track their way to you.

I tell people about the Red Tent by saying it's a held safe space where everyone gets a chance to speak and be heard, and to just drop into being themselves away from family life and all the rest of it. I don't particularly go into that much detail about it. I think at that point, people will either get it or they'll ask questions about it. I might say it's really friendly, there's no judgement just come as you are, and it's all confidential. Because I think that's what people worry about: Is it going to be safe for me? Am I going to be judged? So I would normally emphasise the aspects of it that are more about sister-hood, I guess. I think generally, if someone's wanting that, when you start talking about it they get it straight away, because they're thinking, I know I need that. I don't know what it is but it sounds really good. It's more of a knowing isn't it, then? I think that's probably why I can't always articulate it, because it is more of a knowing than an intellectual thing.

I think the name might be a deterrent too…which is why I didn't use the word Red Tent when I started it, because I thought it might detract from what it was. So I just called it 'women's circle'. But even then, what's a circle? It all needs a bit of explaining to extend inclusion to all women everywhere.

Lily

The invitation needs to hold all the information for the Red Tent to provide a sense of what is expected, the considerations you have made for people to feel welcome and practical information. You can evoke a sense of your Red Tent with the tone and style of language you use and the way you describe what will happen.

Communicating Accessibility

Part of addressing accessibility is to be clear about who is welcome and naming them when you promote and publicise your Red Tent. Clarity is a way to avoid indirect exclusion or assumptions about who is *welcome* and who is *other*. The experience of being othered is often an act of not being seen.

For example, if you are at an event where everyone is invited to make their way up the stairs into the main hall and you use a wheelchair to get around, then that 'everyone' will not include you, and you may need to ask where the lift is. It may be met with helpful information or an awkward explanation about the lift being out of action.

It is far better if you are holding a Red Tent to ensure you communicate that there is stair-free access or lifts provided, instead of placing the responsibility on someone who needs them to seek clarification as to whether the event is accessible for them. Clarity is one important step in helping make spaces more accessible.

So in planning your communications about your Red Tent consider each of the issues we reflected on in the 'Liberating Space' section and ask yourself:

★ *How does this consideration affect how you communicate about your Red Tent both outside and within your community?*

★ *What does this consideration make you think you might be missing?*

★ *What opportunities for inclusion and promoting equity in your Red Tent can you see when you consider this?*

A few of us from different women's circles and organisations co-developed a trans women welcome logo which could be included on any website and publicity. It was designed by a woman artist who is trans and any donations for its use go to support work with young trans people. People have said they only felt safe to come because of this symbol letting them know they would be welcome.

Clare

Creating your invite

Making a template to use for each month is a helpful way to ensure you have included everything you want to say and have an agreed language and approach to inviting people to your Red Tent. Some helpful aspects to include are:

★ a short description about what a Red Tent is and your shared vision for its place in your community;

★ a clear sense of who is welcome and what provisions have been made or are offered to make it feel open and accessible. For example, make it explicit that this gathering is for all cis and trans women, as well as non-binary people who are comfortable in a space that is female-of-centre. As Persia said to us, "If it says you're welcome as a trans woman, I know I am.";

★ the practical information like timings for arrival and departure and anything else that feels relevant. If someone is unsure about attending a particular Red Tent then they may appreciate having a more extensive explanation about the process and way of doing things in the group – "This happens and then we do this…";

★ the details of where it is and directions, including relevant information about parking and public transport;

★ whether there is a maximum number of women able to attend the space and if there is a reserve list and how that will operate;

★ if there is a request or invitation for women to bring something to share, wear something red and food or refreshment;

✱ always include contacts details and what you need from people to limit additional questions and admin on your part.

When we talk about safer spaces what we are talking about is spaces that are made safer because of the parameters that we put in place. This is integral to Red Tents as we want everyone to show up and feel able to receive what they need.

Aisha

Online

There are many simple tools used to organise community events, held spaces and supportive connections online. Knowing your audience locally is crucial. Most people organise Red Tents using online ways to contact people alongside word of mouth and some posters or notices in their communities. During the Covid-19 pandemic, with many Red Tents operating online, technology is being used to hold as well as to advertise Red Tents.

The Red Tent Directory is of course one way to share your Tent online! But in addition to listing with us, you may decide to create a mailing list, website or a social media presence or all three! Some women use an event listing site to promote their events and have women sign up or register through them. Many Tents have their own social media groups or pages while others may have a simple website.

When we have our meetings, we tend to arrange them online between the organisers first, and then we put out advertisements to what we offer through Facebook and Instagram. We have also created flyers and posters to put around local areas, in places such as local libraries, charity shops and anywhere else that will let us. Word of mouth is always helpful, and we always encourage people that come to a Red Tent to think of any of their friends who might enjoy or benefit from coming to bring them along too. We encourage active participation in the online groups as this can make people feel that they know each other somewhat, making meeting in real life less intimidating. Sharing information about other groups, news, and any other interesting articles online creates a feeling of community and togetherness.

Michelle

Having a virtual method for inviting people to your Red Tent is probably the best way to stay organised and consistent, as well as to make it easy for people to share about the Red Tent with other women they know. Sending out an email invitation is easier if you create a multiple contact group in your email account or if you are feeling a little more adventurous, you could create an email account just for your Red Tent. Eventually, if your Tent grows you may have to limit numbers at each meeting.

We've got 500 on the Facebook group and about 350 on a mailing list for twenty places at each Red Tent and so sometimes we have a waiting list. Some are super keen and come to almost every meeting and then we have quite a lot of people who come when they can, and we have a few people who come twice a year. So, it's really quite a mix. There's definitely a core of regulars every time, so even if there's five newbies, they come into something that's established. I think you can really relax when you're just joining into what's already structured. They feel they can just join in the flow.

Lou and Laura

Confidentiality

The important thing about your email list is confidentiality and consent for how you will use the names and addresses that you have been given. It is important to be sensitive to people's details so that they are not used for other purposes. From our experience, it is also good at an early stage to agree how often and what you will communicate to people, keeping it related to Red Tents and not using it to promote other work or workshops.

Be sure not to allow people's email addresses to be visible to all the other recipients when sending out group emails by putting your own email address in the 'To' box, and placing all the recipients in the 'BCC' box. Ensure that your computer and the services that you use to contact people are as secure as possible and that paper records of people's emails and phone numbers are also kept secure and confidential, and that you do not pass on contact details without express permission.

Dress Code

Many Tents invite women to show up wearing something red to symbolise shared connection, and the sense of a feminine energy that some Red Tents seek to celebrate. It provides a way of connecting immediately to each other if we share the same colour palette when we arrive. You can also think of it as putting on something intentional to enter a different kind of space from our day-to-day routine. Many women choose to dress up...others choose comfort and warmth that they don't get to experience in their daily work clothes. There is no one right way to do this but you might choose to provide guidance on this in the invitation.

REFLECTIVE QUESTIONS

★ How will you invite people to and promote your Tent?

★ In what ways can you be clear about accessibility and inclusion in your publicity?

★ What words will you use to speak to women's hunger for these spaces?

★ What qualities of the Red Tent do you think are most important?

★ What ways can you convey unplanned space for connection simply and succinctly?

★ What tools will you use to carry your message?

★ Which forms of 'getting the word out' feel most nourishing and easy for you?

★ What are the most essential parts of a Red Tent that you want to convey when you describe it?

★ Where, if at all, do you feel stretched by this and who and how might you ask for help?

Finances and Resourcing Your Tent

Finance is probably the topic we have had the most questions and discussions about over the past eight years at the Red Tent Directory. And so, we think it is important that you agree as a group how you will handle money and donations from the outset.

We believe that Red Tents can be spaces that challenge the current economic paradigm and that the co-creation that can emerge from holding to the principle of free or donation-based Tents can both sustain and grow a different kind of community space. Indeed, we think Red Tents can be an example of practicing a different model of resourcing, but for this to be possible we have to be clear with one another if doubts and questions start to emerge.

At the Red Tent Directory our listing policy states that we list gatherings which are either free or donation-based, with donations used to cover the cost of room hire or tea and with the amount of the donation ideally being left to the discretion of the donor. Free or donation-based Tents help promote access for *all* women, and this, in and of itself, is core to the purpose of Red Tents. They also challenges the idea that Red Tents are another workshop or business opportunity.

Keeping our Tents free of promotion of our work of any kind and making sure that they were always free was such an important principle for us at the Brighton Red Tent. I feel it has greatly contributed to the longevity and health of our community. There are so many places where we can promote ourselves especially in a therapy-strong town like Brighton, so the Red Tent was a sacred place where any outward identities we may hold were left at the door and this was really valuable to us.

Jill

The vision we hold is for spaces created in the community by a group of women and open to all. To us accessibility means doing all we can to make a Red Tent that any woman in your community is welcome to attend. This also means not making the cost prohibitive to any woman, and therefore donations being of a flexible amount depending on circumstances.

We ask for a non-compulsory donation and if there's any extra money we use that towards buying candles, tissues, essences, massage oils, herbs and recently some padded pop-up chairs. We have had people with various physical issues and pop-up chairs (sometimes known as backjacks) are great for those who need a bit more support.
Laura and Lou

We think of Red Tents as an extension of what we might do in other friendships in our lives. And so, just as we wouldn't charge our friends for our support in a time of crisis, nor do we charge for a Red Tent.

I am a strong advocate of a Red Tent being like a smile, a smile has no price, so it should be free... If you pay for it, it is really not the same!
Yanick

We believe that Red Tents can be nurtured by a group of women working together to hold and create community. That together we can develop an understanding of what it means to share leadership of these spaces, as distinct from how it feels to run a business offering for women, as many of us do in the rest of our lives.

We also know that, living in a capitalist economic system and society, the idea of Red Tents being something that is part of a business structure, is out there. But we believe that the way in which we have been thinking about Red Tents as a radical cultural act is better supported in alternative and co-created ways. We have also, over time, noticed that it is the Tents held by a group of women that tend to be more sustainable, both for the people holding them and the community in general than those run by an individual as an add-on to their other business activities.

Of course, where there are costs associated with holding a Red Tent, for example, contributing to the cost of a venue, receiving donations is a reasonable way of covering those. This is not about women being out of pocket or forcing people into great personal cost that they don't share. Rather, we hope that women will share responsibility for co-creating Red Tents so that the burden is shared and the experience is a nourishing one for *all* women involved. That's why we support donation-based spaces where they feel appropriate. Within this framework, Red Tents approach money and donations in a variety of different ways.

The Red Tent Directory itself is something we have created as a free listing space and, over the years it has be growing, we have chosen to invest our own time and resources in it. Whilst we are now beginning to ask for donations and offer some resources at a small cost to support its upkeep, we never intend to make the support and information we provide something out of which any of us make a profit. For us, this is a sacred principle with this work, though of course, it challenges us at times. We live in a culture where charging for things is the norm and where sharing our homes, experiences, food and times with others, particularly with women we don't yet know, can feel counter-cultural.

Having said all of this, all of us involved in the Directory make money in the world in other ways, including offerings for women which may, on the face of it seem similar to this space. We are not against women generating an income in any way. It is important for us to earn a livelihood. But we have viewed this work as community building and culture building and so have continued to resource it even through periods without work, during our maternity leave and whilst working abroad, leaning into one another when we can and need to take time and space for ourselves. It is because we are doing it together that we are able to do this.

Our suggestion, therefore, is that you ask for contributions if you incur costs in holding your Red Tent. For example, for the venue or to cover anything that you buy to help create it, and that as far as you can you ask women to donate whatever is required to help your Red Tent exist and grow. For example, you might ask women to bring or donate decorations, food to share before or during your Red Tent, and items to support any creative activities which you plan to do or that they may wish to share.

Promotions within your Red Tent

You may find that issues of money and the promotion of services come to the surface and need to be addressed within your Red Tent. Often some of the women who help to hold and attend Red Tents have related offerings that they do charge for, either as a practitioner or as part of a business they run or work for. Sometimes, indeed, you may be asked to, or feel that you want to, promote these offerings.

However, if your invitations or circles become focused on one or more other offerings, we have found that this can detract from the spirit and intention of the Red Tent which is – for us, at least – about creating a shared, open space for all. We suggest, therefore, that you consider finding a way to do this that doesn't interfere with the intention or main space of your Red Tent. Obviously we don't want to prevent women from sharing their skills and talents and discourage them from making a living, but in our experience it is best to keep both the invitations and communications about the Red Tent and the sharing during the circle itself free from promotion, advertising or services. Women are then of course free to share about their work and offerings during social time or perhaps you may wish to provide a special place for that sharing at the end of your Red Tents or through another form of connection between the women who attend them.

REFLECTIVE QUESTIONS

★ How do you feel about money and your Tent?

★ What costs do you or will you have? How could you share them with the women who will co-hold and attend your Tent?

★ What culture of money and resources do you want to create in your Red Tent community?

★ How does this align with your values and the values of the space you will create?

7.

LEADERSHIP

What do we mean by leadership? This book is about community held and run Red Tents and so, by leadership we definitely don't mean doing everything yourself, making all the plans or telling everyone what to do.

We want to invite you to think about an alternative sort of leadership, different to the kind we usually see modelled in the world today where a single heroic leader is in charge and leads from the front.

We believe in – and want to invite you into – a model of leadership where we commit to being in the practice of walking our talk. This means that we strive in the way in which we lead, and how we understand leadership, to embody and practice the things that we are promoting and inviting through the whole idea and vision of Red Tents as collectively held and anti-oppressive structures.

What does this specifically mean when we set out to run Red Tents? For us, it means being in the practice of caring for ourselves, taking time for ourselves and also, since we believe in community held and run Tents, being in the practice of sharing leadership and space with other women.

We also want to acknowledge that not everyone we have interviewed for this book runs their Red Tent in a collective model. Some women we have interviewed for this book have found other ways to build support for themselves whilst running a Red Tent. They have learnt to care for themselves with clear boundaries, self-care practices and a group of close friends for support so that they are able to offer their energy to the holding of the Red Tent alone.

For ourselves, we have explored what it means to do this collectively in the way that we have run the Red Tent Directory website, sharing leadership of the project with each other from the beginning: speaking up when things are too much, taking a break when we need to and honouring one another's needs as we work together on the project. We have tried to embody and share these values with the other women who have volunteered to support the Directory over the past eight years. We don't always live up to this when it's hard, and when we don't manage, we try again. We keep holding the vision of the kind of leadership we want to see in the world and experience around us and we try to live it into being. So something we want to invite you to think about is: *how do you want to embody the values of your Red Tent in the way in which you hold, create and lead it?*

Red Tents offer us the opportunity to dismantle our conditioning of hier-archical leadership models. If we are to avoid burn out, create safe spaces for our inner work, and fully step into our power as women, we urgently need to adopt our authentic feminine leadership which calls for a shared and collaborative holding of space [in which] we never go it alone, we always call in support! We have a responsibility to explore our relation-ship to leadership and authority to understand how and what we project onto others both as facilitators and participants. It can be shadowy, our wounds are deep here, but this is where the transformation happens.
Cali

The original root of the word 'lead' is associated with causing travel and making movement[1] and so it was more about what you move towards than how you dictate things to others. In relation to Red Tents we think about us collectively leading something we could think about as travel – movement away from the ways in which women have related to each other competi-tively and critically within the structures of patriarchy and moving instead towards a more supportive culture in which our relationships to one another help us, and those around us, to thrive.

But often we can't do this, we can't be in a supportive relationship to one another, unless we are able to acknowledge any sadness and anger about the ways in which we may have struggled with these things in the past. We also

---

1   The root word of leadership is lead from the Anglo-Saxon Old English word 'loedan', the causal form of 'lithan' to travel.
See ila-net.org/Publications/Proceedings/2003/mgrace.pdf

need to be willing to give ourselves support as this kind of leader. In our experience, leading in this way requires us to reject the idea that in order to lead we must always be right, we must always do it our way or we must exhaust ourselves for the cause.

When our relationship to ourselves is one of constant burdening and pushing, when we feel we must always be giving and doing more, we are doing ourselves – in subtle ways – the very same disservice we are so committed to preventing for others. We are neglecting our basic human needs.

Mary Ann [2]

We think instead about the personal and collective structures that can support us to be effective leaders of *travel towards* a more supportive culture amongst women being modelled in Red Tent spaces, a culture that we believe can also have a positive impact on those around us, on the world. Here are some of the things we have found useful for this:

★ care practices that we honour for ourselves as well as monthly as part of the Tent, such as rest, taking time out, doing things we love…;

★ learning to say *no*;

★ building a collective structure of support for ourselves as leaders;

★ developing group leadership structures for Red Tents that support us to lead together;

★ doing our own work to deal with emotional issues and challenges;

★ acknowledging our sadness and anger and all the feelings and emotions that come up;

★ **staying reflective** and experiential about the structures and processes – in other words, learning as we go!

2   This is from a blog Mary Ann wrote: how-matters.org/2017/06/21/how-we-treat-ourselves

Group Leadership Structures for Red Tents

I, Aisha, have a hidden Wonder Woman costume in my wardrobe which gets a fair bit of dusting off these days! You might know the feeling? It's the metaphorical costume I put on when I'm balancing holding responsibility for caring for my family, work priorities and the rest of my life, including supporting friends as they struggle with what they are holding too! Sounds like too much, right? And at times it is. But it doesn't need to be like this in everything we do. The Red Tent is an opportunity to co-create a structure where there is space to lead, room to listen and ways to share decision-making.

Leadership in a community recognises that there are many ways of showing up. Let's look at a few different approaches we might need to enable us to hold responsibility with others. We think of these as different perspectives and energies that we each might bring, perhaps at different times, to the holding of our Red Tent circles.

★ **Clarity** – The energy that gets issues discussed and decisions made by being vocal and direct. This might be sharing about the Tent or co-holding meetings so that they have some process and direction.

★ **Collective** – Leading by being alongside is about supporting each other to take things forward. This looks like making shared decisions and finding ways to compromise and seeking to resolve conflict.

★ **Nurturing** – Leading 'from behind' is about supporting others to use their initiative, either by training them up or instilling confidence in their ability. This might involve supporting others and encouraging them to do things.

★ **Visionary** – Leading by taking a step back means you can see the bigger picture and the implications for the wider community. This part is where we strategise and take a longer view. It can also be the part where we lead by getting out of the way!

Many women who want to set up a Red Tent or help in running one are doing so because they want the support that Red Tents offer and the opportunity to let go of their everyday roles and responsibilities. Given this, one of the benefits of a community-led Red Tent is that it enables things to happen, without one person feeling that they always have to be up front leading it all. In this way everyone can benefit from the space as well as helping to co-create it.

Power

Power can be conceptualised as energy that can be used in whatever way we choose. Sharing leadership means intentionally sharing power. It understands that 'power over' others is just one way in which power can be felt and expressed in the world. Another way to think about power is to consider this analysis of power offered by Lisa VeneKlasen in which she frames four different types of power:[3]

★ our own 'Power Within';

★ the 'Power To' which we have and can use to take action;

★ the 'Power With' we can generate together;

★ 'Power Over' (where we dominate others – a kind we see a lot in the world but want to be cautious of in Red Tent spaces).

We can orientate our framework for holding structures for Red Tents around coming together to generate 'Power With' by capitalising on our own 'Power Within' and 'Power To'. In other words, to make sure we are practicing our own care and support as we have described and to support one another to take creative action as we create our Red Tents in the world.

The holding circle

In this book we use this term to describe a monthly circle of women coming together to plan a Red Tent, make decisions together and share a collective to-do list. A structure like this enables many women to contribute to running the Red Tent and ensuring its long-term sustainability. Some Red Tents we have interviewed for this book choose another name for a very similar structure. The holding circle is created to share a collective responsibility and acts as a place for the wider community to feed in ideas and contribute to the running and organising of the Red Tent. By coming together in physical space or as an online group, it is possible to talk through tasks, share challenges, and ask for help. In between these meet ups, discussions can take place between those in the holding circle, as long as the bigger decisions are shared in the wider circle gatherings. It is also a fun way of getting things done, rather than slipping on that personal Wonder Woman costume and staying up late to finish things off when you need to sleep!

In the circle space I have witnessed shifts for those sharing their pain and seen wisdom being exchanged through both tears and laughter. These profound moments often hinge on women who are running circles and their ability to hold the space.

Madeleine

There isn't a magic formula for creating collective holding structures and we can't promise the perfect formula or an approach that is certain to have no bumps in the road. However, we do have some pointers for you which are built from what we have learned ourselves and from the women we have interviewed for this book:

★ develop a culture of stepping up to lead. By stepping up, others get to step back, so it is nourishing for everyone. By stepping up, you get to feel a part of something growing and evolving. By stepping up you learn new things about yourself and others;

★ create a journey to leadership – ask people how they would like to contribute and encourage them as sometimes people feel hesitant about offering;

★ write simple guides to doing things so you don't assume knowledge about how to do things and then later wish you had offered more guidance;

★ draw in additional support – ask people to help who have specific skills to assist with relevant tasks;

★ plan for what happens when life gets in the way – ways to ease or share the burden or approaches to people stepping out and then stepping in again later;

★ expect to learn, have problems, explore them, apologise or make amends, forgive and learn again;

★ manage expectations and try to resolve issues within the community as they arise;

★ think about the support and reflection your group needs to be able to show up and hold space for the Red Tent effectively and to make it true that everyone is welcome;

★ sometimes an unforeseen challenge that one person has can create space to enable others to step up and hold a Red Tent or take on a new role. This is the beauty of adapting to what arises in the moment both within the community and the wider world.

Ingrid, who offered to run the virtual Tent, lives alone. She felt called to run a virtual circle at the start of the pandemic, specifically for women who are also living alone, or are single. It was organised as an hour online with a "cup of tea to keep us warm as we won't have the physical warmth of each other". Space was offered for five women on a first-come first-served basis (although in the end twelve responded and were all given a place!) Each woman had space to check in uninterrupted as well as an opportunity to check out, offering gratitude for something. Other virtual circles are now being offered to women who live with others as well. Incredibly, all of these new virtual circles have been offered by different women in the North London Red Tent Community, some of whom have participated in Red Tents but never 'held' one before. They have felt able to 'step up' here with the support of a telephone call from one of the elders of the community. The circles have been rich and supportive.
Mads

For some groups that cover a larger region, with many caretakers or where people travel large distances, it may make more sense to hold the holding circles online, as travelling twice a month to meet may not be feasible.

Collective Decision-Making and Hidden Hierarchy

We want to highlight the fact that making collective decisions is not always easy, and that the circle as a structure is not a panacea. Unspoken hierarchies and conflicts can still manifest within structures that are intended to be collaborative or co-operative. Living in housing co-ops, Aisha witnessed that the hierarchies and power dynamics often replicate themselves in collective spaces, even when our expressed intention is to dismantle them. We have both experienced this in other spaces too. When this happens, we are falling into what Ella Scheepers and Ishtar Lakhani have called the "form trap". As they point out: "The choice to adopt a horizontal structure (or to hold a particular form for a meeting) with the intention of creating an open, non-hierarchical, and inclusive space, may not necessarily produce the intended effect. In fact, it may end up as nothing more than a performance of equality or inclusivity or some other social purpose goal (Nilsson 2015), but the opposite is experienced by those in the room. This is because power can operate invisibly and even unconsciously (Lukes 2005). Once the form is in place, it gives the appearance of commitment to the goal, but it is symbolic rather than real…even the most horizontally structured organisation or the most 'inclusive' meeting can be as silencing and violent, no matter what its 'form' looks like from the outside."[3]

If the group is willing and able to acknowledge any hierarchies that are present and be as transparent as possible about them, then this challenge can be explored and help build the actual potential for collective decision-making. It sometimes helps to acknowledge that there are natural hierarchies in place even in a space that is apparently collective. Perhaps some of those present bring many years of experience and are respected for their experience or commitment, maybe they are the initiator of an idea in the first place. Rather than pretending everyone is equal in the space, instead we suggest that you name it, talk about it and work with it consciously and intentionally.

For example, in the Red Tent Directory, all the team involved take part in the decisions we make, but it would be unhelpful if we (Aisha and Mary Ann) didn't acknowledge that both as founders and having seen the many years of ebb and flow of the project, that our voices are important. We

---

3 "Caution! Feminists at work: building organizations from the inside out," Ella Scheepers and Ishtar Lakhani, from *Gender and Development*, vol 28, no1, Reimagining International Development, Edited by Mary Ann Clements and Caroline Sweetman

have realised that it is disingenuous to assume we can have collective decision-making on everything we do. Understandably, members of the team often want to know what we think first, before challenging it, agreeing or offering alternatives. And so now we attempt to own that hierarchy and admit that it is present in a way that allows others to challenge and disagree with us, but also to lean on us for support.

Collective leadership structures then can be used in all kinds of ways. It is important, when using a shared holding circle to run a Red Tent space, to be clear about the intentions and have clarity about the principles. What is important is not to let the form of a *circle* become, as Sheepers and Lakhani put it, "symbolic rather than experiential". In other words, if we want leadership to genuinely be shared, we need to keep paying attention to the dynamics and feelings we are actually experiencing while at the same time welcoming them into our awareness so we can continually reflect together on the ways in which we are working. In this way, the circle structure, which we talk more about later in the book, and the process of speaking and actively listening to each other can support the group. It can enable many opinions to be raised, issues to be discussed without being closed down and for feelings to be owned around the group.

Some of them had never held space before for a circle of women. They'd done a lot of different things in their own roles and jobs, and you can see the difference between the ones who started four years ago and how they are now. It's just amazing, and that's credit to them as well, because they've taken on board what and how we do things, and then decided, maybe that's not me, I'll do this my way. So there's a structure, but there's also flexibility.
Lou and Laura

Another aspect of the holding circle structure is the opportunity for more members of the Red Tent community to step up and take on roles. One way of making people feel welcome is by letting them feel that they can contribute to making Red Tents happen. If you meet in a different woman's house each time, then asking new women to host a Red Tent in their home is one way to involve them. Moving the gatherings shares this role around. If you meet in the same community space, dance studio or outdoor venue, then asking different women to help set up, decorate the venue and pack things away are also ways to involve them.

Accountability in a Group

An important element of collective leadership is being accountable to the group for tasks that you have agreed to. If we don't keep the commitments we make to one another then collective leadership cannot function effectively. When you agree to do something, we envisage it as if you have taken the task out of the group space and you are literally holding it in your hands. It is perhaps an obvious point, but if, for whatever reason, you cannot fulfil this role or do the thing you have offered to complete, then you need to hold yourself accountable within the group. This might be by explaining why you haven't done it and proposing a way to make sure it gets completed by another person or with a different approach. Being clear about what you have and haven't done in this way is what makes you reliable, resourceful and helps you to release any potential of shame, guilt or struggle.

A thing that we did in the Steering Circle is be honest: if you can't do something, there's no shame if you come forward and say that you can't do a particular task. There's no shame with saying yes, or no or maybe, not if we're walking our talk.

Elaine

The alternative is that you feel you have let down the group and perhaps yourself too. The manifestations of this is often that it sits, festers and delays action completely because you haven't communicated clearly and so these feelings remain unvoiced, unseen and unresolved. From the group perspective the task is incomplete and there is a sense of waiting to know where it is and when it will be done. This time lag can impact others in the group and impinge on their ability to fulfil the tasks that they are holding as well. What may have begun as one task not being completed can escalate to a number of tasks being held in limbo. When group accountability is not upheld then time is wasted, frustration builds and there is stagnancy to the natural flow of things. Ultimately collective leadership is about learning alongside each other about being open about commitments and expectations as you navigate this journey together. Kindness, forgiveness and being honest help support collective leadership to thrive.

We hold a core belief, "All of You is Welcome Here." As we went along, I started to understand that in order to be able to say this meaningfully I have to be able to welcome all parts of myself. This is always going to be work in progress. Nobody is shadow-free and we are likely to have some judgements running in our minds. That's why, I believe, it's helpful, to hold one another as a group. I may be triggered when listening to a woman, perhaps because I haven't been able to welcome the part of myself that she is displaying. But there may be another woman in the circle who has welcomed that part of herself and therefore can hold the energy of compassion in this situation that I'm not yet ready to hold. Having a team plugs the gaps. The circle can more truthfully embody, "All of you is welcome," because you've got that group consciousness, rather than just one individual leader.

Lou

Lou clearly articulates the reason why women who are holding Red Tents need to be in an active practice of self-reflection and discovery and why it was something they focused on in their holding circle. The practice helps them to genuinely welcome women to their Red Tent and also to deal with and process many of the conflicts and issues that come up there. We will look further at conflicts and processing our own challenges later in the book.

Building a Structure of Support for us as Leaders

We have lived through a good half century of individualistic linear organising (led by charismatic individuals or budget building institutions), which intends to reform or revolutionise society; but falls back into modelling the oppressive tendencies against which we claim to be pushing.

adrienne maree brown [4]

---

4   brown, adrienne maree. *Emergent Strategy: Shaping Change, Changing Worlds*

Leadership is often seen as a tough solo role that involves some level of fighting to stay at the top and a strong ego to reinforce any decisions made and protect what you have and hold off those that might want to crush you. But this approach is often lonely and unsustainable. It can create an environment in which it is almost impossible to admit mistakes because there is so much invested in the one single 'hero' figurehead. As we write, we see this manifest in our wider world in relation to the pandemic, to politics, to struggles for racial equality and to almost every aspect of our lives.

To be resilient in the face of challenges and flexible enough to change it is important to lean out into the wise approaches of others, balance ideas with diverse viewpoints and draw on the resources of a wider community. One thing we think about for ourselves, as leaders in many of the things we do in our lives – including the Red Tent Directory – is what are our personal support structures? Who are the people who have our backs? This could be people we are working with, who are part of the holding circle, but often it may also be other people in our lives who we know we can call on when we need help, love and support. There are different types of support[5] we find helpful to consider:

★ people who can help us to think and strategise;

★ people who can give us unfailing positivity and support;

★ people who can energise us and encourage us to be brave;

★ people who can help us have clear boundaries as we say no and encourage us to stay clear and committed to our focus.

We can all benefit from a range of different kinds of support when we are working to make a difference in the world. Establishing your Red Tent is no exception and it is helpful to think about where we might individually draw on the support of sisters. This could come from your Red Tent holding circle, women who run Red Tents elsewhere or people who you know in other parts of your life.

---

5   This framework draws on the archetypes model used in Shadow Work in which Mary Ann is a certified Coach. This in turn draws on Jungian analysis, which in turn borrowed, without due credit, ideas and concepts from Indigenous peoples. We honour the named and unnamed influences on this work.

My experience of going to my women's group had always been one of reassurance and a sense of belonging and acceptance from my sisters. I felt very sure that I could arrive with whatever was moving in me and not have to pretend or perform to be accepted. I would always leave feeling glad I had gone. If I were having a bad day, there was never any need for apology or explanation. If I were having a great day, I could show up like that, without need to make myself small or check myself. All my energy was always welcome.

Su

Think about creating your own personal circle of support that can have your back as you create a Red Tent space for other women. Who do you want to be a part of it? Once you have identified people who can help you in each of the four ways we identify above, get really specific, consider:

★ *Why have you chosen the person and how would you like them to help you?*

★ *Do you want to directly communicate this request for support to them and if so, how will you do so?*

★ *What will you ask them to be available for or to do?*

I find it so helpful to share my thoughts and feelings as it helps me clarify and explore them, and to receive some empathic feedback. It is so enriching to hear others and learn and benefit from the warmth of giving and receiving support.

Clare

Creating a support circle for ourselves in this way can be useful in anything we want to do. You may not ever have all these women together in a room (or you may call them together) but having a virtual circle of women as you work on something in your life can be an invaluable support and resource.

Agreements, Boundaries and Principles

There were boundaries and structure, but they were transparent and they were in place for everyone to help get the work done in the steering circle, because there was a lot of work. I believe that we held true to maintaining those boundaries and it created the safe container for the wider community. Because we were not just in the steering circle together, but we were in the Red Tent together as well. And so therefore, we saw each other in different vulnerabilities, in tears and different moods and expressing different parts of our personality and aspects of ourselves.
Elaine

The establishment and communication of clear agreements is key to building a strong group and leadership. When we say 'agreements' we mean both literal agreements – rules, inclusion, what time the doors open and close – in the shared space which you are creating when you host a Red Tent, as well as personal agreements about how you interact with each other and what you choose to say *yes* and *no* to.

When I, Mary Ann, first learnt about healing spaces that had principles and even rules that governed them, I felt so resistant. My whole life up to that point had been about pushing boundaries and seeking freedom from rules! But what I learnt over time, through experiencing spaces which were organised by a set of simple agreements, was that there was freedom in the simple clarity where everyone present knows what to expect and what the principles of the space are. If we have a clear idea of the kind of space, sometimes called the container, we are seeking to create in our Red Tent gathering and are able to share that with everyone present, then we in fact invite freedom within that structure by giving it some boundaries.

Container

Just like a cup is a container that holds liquid from spilling out, the word 'container' is used in a therapeutic space or group environment to suggest that the mix of energy, personalities, stories and behaviour is held in a vessel to avoid messy splashing and spilling over. It describes the act of establishing parameters within a group so that everyone knows what is expected of them and each other. A container is created to allow a feeling of known safety based on a balance between structure and freedom. It means that participants can speak and listen with awareness. By agreeing on what is welcome it is also suggesting what isn't welcome, that by stepping into this container you are acting with intention. It is created as a temporary holding that has an end, however some of the agreements established may continue outside of this space, such as confidentiality. The idea of a container originates from Indigenous cultures who have known how to create spaces for rituals and communal processing. We honour that legacy though we do not know all of the specific details of it.

For the many years that we have run the Red Tent Directory we have received requests for help and advice. When something tricky happens, and those involved in Red Tents want another opinion or to test out some ways of resolving it, we have been there to help, either with messages back and forth, or on the end of the phone. Many times we have found ourselves reflecting, alongside the person seeking support, about what boundaries might need to be clearly held or what agreements need to be articulated or re-articulated to prevent the conflict or challenge from happening again.

Rather than conceiving of this as a way to exclude or blame people, we think of it as being about building strong foundations for a solid structure for Red Tents and the fact that these challenges are coming up is often a sign that we are learning as we go. If we need to take down a wall to build it anew with what we have learnt, then it may protect us more effectively from the storms that may appear in the future. The opposite to being clear in a Red

Tent is the kind of vagueness about shared culture and practice that can lead to uncomfortable explanations about 'how we do things here'. This is part of what can make some feel unwelcome in our spaces. At its worst when we assume that people know *how we do things around here* without explicitly explaining, there can be blame and shaming when something happens outside of these unspoken assumptions.

For example, if most women present in a circle know that the check-in part of the Red Tent at the beginning is five minutes for each woman to they will take this time as a shared understanding. But if a new person coming to their first Red Tent doesn't know this and speaks twice as long during this time others present might make judgements about them taking up too much space, or claiming more time. In fact, the person simply didn't have the full information. Once this is explained, a perfectly fair response would be, "If only you'd told me!" It may seem a simple thing but that is why we advocate for sharing clear agreements, rather than making assumptions and having to spend a lot of time unpacking misunderstandings and having lengthy chats and apologies.

I remember us being incredibly boundaried, like having these kind of rules. And we were creating these boundaries so that we wouldn't have potential conflicts in the future. Really it seems mad, but that's why we held them so clearly. Having a clear way of doing things gave me a sense of safety in the Red Tent. We wrote down what happened in the welcome part, the first check-in, the second check-in... We got really clear that this is a structure that we're working towards. By walking the talk, women trusted us. And by me feeling in my body and trusting that I could share my vulnerability, whether in the Steering Circle or the Red Tents, was because of all the work that we actually put in there in the background.
Elaine

Honouring Personal Boundaries

Boundaries are the distance at which I can love myself and you simultaneously.
Prentis Hemphill [6]

At the root of strong group agreements, are healthy personal boundaries. We cannot have one without the other. And so, as we reflect on this topic, we invite you to think more generally about how boundaries show up in your own life and the lives of those around you.

How do you make choices about what you do and don't do in your own life?

Do you have clarity about what you do or don't want? Is there anything that feels difficult in relation to that clarity for you?

How are women who say 'no', or are clear about what they want, viewed in our cultures?

At its simplest, lacking boundaries means not being able to say no. This shows up in our society at every level. In a culture where sexual abuse and sexism have been normalised for generations, many women have learnt in so many ways that saying no and standing up for ourselves is not acceptable, and may even be dangerous. This doesn't just show up in response to direct or indirect abuse, it's around us in the cultural soup we are swimming in, and so it also shows up in our expectations of ourselves and of one another. For example, we may have learnt that good girls don't make a fuss or that saying no is selfish.

For many of us, having clarity about what we want to say yes to in our lives may also have become difficult. In Mary Ann's experience she found that she had to learn to say *no* – something she had really struggled with in the past – before she could get clear about what she actually wanted to say *yes* to. A deep habit of saying *yes* to almost everything had made it difficult, over the years, to discern what she actually wanted to say a big and clear *yes* to, as well as what she didn't want to agree to. This can show up as compulsive volunteering, saying *yes* to all the opportunities that come before us, always feeling we must be the one to help or fix things, as well as an inability

6   *Finding Our Way* podcast with Prentis Hemphill, "Episode 2 – Visioning with adrienne maree brown"

to say *no* to abusive or manipulative situations in our lives.

On some level, we believe that we all want to be loved…while at the same time many of us feel like we are somehow not enough to be loved as we are. This deeply rooted sense of being innately inadequate sometimes shows up in our desire to do a million things and be a thousand different personas to suit every situation. Aisha identifies with this helping and rescuing narrative and has in the past often found herself working full time for a charity while volunteering for a number of other projects and campaigns at the same time. It took a total burnout for her to realise that, yes she may believe in a multitude of causes, however, the tireless desire to give of herself in order to feel worthy is not healthy.

Sometimes we become so fixated on offering a valuable contribution that benefits others, that we ignore our own needs. Somewhere within us this can come from a messy mix of wanting love and feeling alone: emotions that are best served with a bit of fresh air and a hug, so that when you do show up for a cause, campaign or phone call you can do so from a more resourced place. Everything we do fulfils a need, it is about finding the balance of what serves you, and serves others at the same time, and not unravelling in the process.

Expending ourselves is an expectation of our cultures and the way they often seem to value women being busy and doing it all. And in response we often find that we over-serve and derive value from *being useful,* being a *good girl* and saying *yes* to everything. This is one way that we enact patriarchy on ourselves and so by encouraging one another to have boundaries and choose deliberately, we are supporting one another to resist this.

In the Red Tent we want to invite you to consciously think about creating clear boundaries as an antidote to a culture in which many of us say *yes* because we always say *yes.* A culture where women saying *yes* to caring, looking after, birthing and nurturing, has been relied upon and exploited, and in which women saying *yes* to lower wages and being treated as second-class citizens has also, historically been the norm. Probably, for most of us, we are currently saying *yes* to things that we would like, given half a chance, to say *no* to. We may not always be able to scramble for that *no.* We may need to keep saying *yes* right now. However, when it comes to choosing how we want to give our time to community movements, volunteer opportunities or campaigns for empowering women, is there a way that we can dip our toe into saying *yes* and *no* to the right things for us?

Can we learn through our relationships together what lights us up or turns us off?

Is there a way that women can be sparring partners for one another to help us all develop more healthy boundaries, so that when it really matters for the big things we have some practice under our belt and can choose with power and integrity?

Over the years of running a number of teams of volunteers and organisations, we have learnt that we would also actually prefer people to gift us with their *no* rather than mess us around with their *yes*. There is nothing worse than someone saying *yes* when they don't have capacity, and then a slow painful exchange ensues where we chase them, encourage, motivate and support them to take action, before they finally tell us they don't have the time right now to take on the challenge. This wastes everyone's time and energy and brings us back to offering you the idea of the sheer beauty of knowing where someone's boundaries lie. Not only do you know what to expect from them, but you know how to manage your own gifts and limitations around them. If you can gracefully say *no*, you will offer an opportunity to another person who is hungry to take on a new challenge and has the time to do so. In other words, your *no* can be – and usually is – someone else's blessing.

We also want to note that this experience of very often saying *yes* is not the reality for every woman. For some, saying *yes* may be a stretch. You might have got very used to saying *no* as a way to protect yourself, for example, and find that it keeps you safe. That may work brilliantly for you or you may do it even when you really want to say *yes*. Boundaries show up differently for each of us. Saying anything other than *no* might open up a chink in your armour. Taking the risk of being vulnerable may feel like plate tectonics shifting dangerously and who wants the earth to move and sway when you are learning to stand up straight? In this circumstance you might want to gravitate towards getting involved by asking questions, feeling into your interest, working alongside someone else and gaining an understanding of what stepping up may involve. A slow but solid way of leaning into a *yes*, that can ease the heart palpitations, is to follow it up with an additional boundary. For example, add a period of time to taking something on as a trial and then review it periodically: "I'll take that on for a month and see how it feels for me and then review," or something similar that is clear for everyone involved.

Earlier in this book we talked about committing to a year or so of monthly gatherings to give time to the ebb and flow of a growing community, but many hands can contribute towards making this happen rather than one person taking it all on. By being clear about who is agreeing to do what, we can create more resilient ways of being together and holding space for each other.

When we say *yes* to being part of the creation of a Red Tent space in our community, it may be that we need to say *no* to something else. For many of us, saying *no* is a challenge. We may have been raised to think that saying *no* was unhelpful or impolite. We may find it awkward or difficult, we may hate to let other people down. At the cultural level, we believe that an environment in which women find it so difficult to say *no* both keeps us too busy to change the system and makes us additionally vulnerable to abuse and harm. But, we have to get comfortable with our *no*, however hard it may seem. For our communities, for ourselves, for our sisters and our daughters.

If you are a person who struggles to say *no* – and as we have shared we definitely wear this badge! – then it can be helpful to remember that there are a plethora of decisions you make every day in which you are effectively saying *no* to something that you don't even think about. When you walk to work the same way you normally walk, you are saying *no* to all the other ways you could get there. They might be longer, more scenic, more dangerous perhaps, but, literally every time you choose to do something in a particular way you are saying *no* to doing it another way.

There are millions of ways you could choose to live your life. You rule most of them out without thinking about them. What you are actually struggling to say *no* to is usually the things other people happen to wave in front of you that aren't – or are no longer – priorities for you. So, practice saying *no*. This will help you to intentionally create space for the Red Tent you want to establish. Be honest with yourself: is there something that you will need to say *no* to if you want to create that space?

Practicing saying *no* is also something you can do with a trusted friend or partner. You might practice it when nothing is at stake and make a fun game of it saying *no* to the other person's polite requests that you help them out in some way and making a point of holding your boundary.

REFLECTIVE QUESTIONS

★ What are your motivations in taking on the things that you do? In what ways might you be more honest with yourself about them?

★ Where do you find it easy to say *yes* in your life?

★ Where do you find it easy to say *no?*

★ How do you get clear about what you do and don't want to be doing?

★ In what ways is this challenging for you?

★ Where in your life do you want to commit to more *yes* or more *no?*

★ How can you initiate conversations about this with other women in your Red Tent or holding circle?

Feeling Safe

If you have women coming regularly to a Red Tent, you may find over time that the sharing amongst them becomes deeper and more personal. Meanwhile, it is also helpful to be clear that there is no compulsion to share. For many of us, sharing things we have never shared before can be risky and feel uncomfortable. It makes sense for most of us to take time to discern whether an environment feels safe enough for us to share more of ourselves in. In order to facilitate this, you can both trust that women will share what feels safe and useful to them, and make the point specifically that women should feel 100% okay with only sharing what feels good for them. This is about inviting every woman attending your Tent to establish a healthy sense of their own safety in the space. This is very different from assuming a space feels safe to them because it feels safe to you.

When we are very fearful about sharing something, this may be a part of us that is preventing us from having the experience of sharing it with other women, of letting it move. But it also may be a wise part of us that knows that this doesn't feel safe, at this point in time, in this place.

Being a small (although geographically widespread) population meant that there were many overlaps in our community. Over time, this meant that we had to navigate various conflicts. For example, one woman going through a divorce whilst another woman became involved with her ex. The woman going through the divorce wanted to use the Red Tent space to express how difficult she was finding the situation and to vent about her ex. The other woman found it difficult to share this space with a woman who was 'bad mouthing' the man she was falling in love with. We had a ritual to state 'all your energy is welcome' at the beginning of each Red Tent. This meant that a container was created and even if a woman was triggered by another, she had already acknowledged that she had welcomed her energy. This puts the responsibility back onto each woman to hold what is their own and hold space for another. This enabled any women in conflict to come back into connection and have compassion for each other.

Su

We can't guarantee the safety of our Red Tent spaces. We can endeavour to create spaces that are well held and offer an opportunity to share and be heard because of our clear agreements. At the same time, each woman must choose for herself what feels right and comfortable for her to share.

We like to say 'safer' spaces to indicate that some ways of intentionally making a space safer have been considered and introduced. Many women describe Red Tents as safe spaces, reflecting their experience of what it is like to be in a gathering like this. It also draws a comparison to less safe shared places, which many of us experience elsewhere. However, we know that it is always possible that women may feel triggered by what others share or by personal interactions in the space and that this may lead to them feeling unsafe, even if there is no actual physical threat in the room.

We all carry a lot with us when we come to a space. As Gwynn Raimondi puts it, "It is about all the past atrocities we have individually experienced and participated in as well as those of our ancestors. We are in a time where all the trauma in our DNA is begging for release".[7] The fact that we now know that trauma can be passed not only through our relationships to our

---

7   medium.com/@gwynnraimondi/these-times-do-not-have-to-be-traumatic-1eeda284bd89

own caregivers but also literally through our biochemistry[8] from generation to generation is just one of the reasons why those who come to Red Tent spaces – and in fact those whom we meet in our lives in other ways – bring so much. They are likely carrying not just their own stories, but also those of their ancestors, which we are now discovering are imprinted on our DNA.

Making spaces trauma-informed can help address some of this and at the same time we cannot take responsibility for everything that turns up in a space. There are gentle ways to invite everyone attending to take responsibility for themselves, which we will share more about later.

Not Therapy

We do believe that there is a positive power in sharing in a community that can feel healing. But, at the same time, Red Tents are deliberately community-led spaces within which we can be heard and seen, *not* spaces to be fixed or to develop therapeutic type relationships. We honour the practitioners that create therapeutic group spaces, but the Red Tent is not this. Rather it is a co-created community space. We don't believe that there is a particular qualification you need to create this kind of container in your community. In fact, we want to invite each and every woman to feel comfortable, and if she would like to, to be someone who holds or takes part in the holding of a Tent.

There are various trainings you can do and initiations into holding Red Tents, but I'm not up for that. I think any woman, every woman, who just follows their intuition can do a Red Tent. There's nothing magic, although it's all magic, but there's no training that you have to do. You don't need to be a counsellor or anything like that, just do it!

Susan

We envisage this kind of space to be widely available to women and to be something any woman can choose to hold and share collectively. Of course, each of us that gets involved in the Red Tent will bring our skills and ex-

---

8   See also Resmaa Menakem who explains this clearly in his book *My Grandmother's Hands: Racialized Trauma and the Pathway to Mending our Hearts and Bodies*

periences with us. But in the Red Tent we consciously lay them down, not because they don't matter – they do – but because we are co-creating a space to be in together without putting on our professional masks, without relying on our qualifications, without needing to be this or that. We are creating a community space where we can show up and share honestly whatever is here for us in the moment.

We're just a witness to whatever women need to share. We are there to try not to judge, although, hands up who judges! I mean we all judge, but let's just watch that judgment and be gentle with that judge. Know that we're doing it and just say, "Leave me alone for the moment. I'll get back to you later. Just shine a light on what we need to heal."
Susan

We are absolutely in favour of professional and non-professional support, therapy, counselling and all the many modalities in which some people in your community may be trained. But we want to invite you to think about the Red Tent being a different kind of space to those that we go to seeking this direct kind of support. Instead, this is a space for us to be together, as equals, to cultivate a way of relating to each other that prioritises being heard and seen and not needing to 'be anyone' or 'fix anyone' or solve anything at all. The Red Tent is a space to rest into. A space just to *be*. We think clear agreements and structures as we have discussed in this section are the tools that help make this type of space possible. They are key to creating a Red Tent that can be held collectively and be sustained.

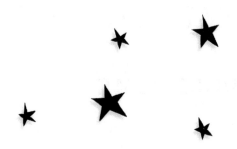

PART THREE

8.

CIRCLE TIME

Hearing other women's stories has helped me to make sense of my own life. As others speak, I recognise myself in them, as if they are giving me a language to understand myself more deeply. It's amazing to have a space to simply 'be', rather than 'do', to relax, and to share tea, cake, laughter, tears and the truth about ourselves.

Ali W

Often our lives are so full of being busy, doing and organising. So far, we've been inviting you to think of Red Tents as an alternative to that; an opportunity to create space to just *be*, let go and go with the flow. But how do you allow and enable that to happen? How do you welcome women in and help them to shift gears?

In this section we describe how we set up and hold the space for the Red Tent, how we welcome each person in, create a container, and establish the circle through ritual and check in.

Preparing the Space

When we started, we put out a lot of decorations and lots of red material, but now I just put a red scarf on the floor and a candle and a talking stick. I think just because it's simpler for me!

Camille

One of the women in the community is a craftswoman and she made us a big wooden hook. We bought a bunch of saris and tied these red and purple and pink saris in a big loop and suspended it from the ceiling, so we had this permanent Red Tent that was always there as a visual symbolic reminder that it was a safe and sacred space.

Emily

There are many different ways to prepare the space for a Red Tent. Some Tents are decorated very simply and just invite women to sit in a circle with a candle in the middle, others are decorated with lots of red materials and objects. However you prepare the space, we encourage you to think about the invitation to sit together, feel connected and share, in the way in which you organise the Red Tent space.

The sumptuous reds and scarlets, the vibrant fabrics and soft fleece, silk and organza. Tapestries adorning walls and cushions and throws on floors and sofas. The transformation of a space from a residential living room into a Red Tent. Meditation, nourishing food, a circle in which to speak and listen, a space to share and to reflect.

Vanessa [1]

Here are some ideas if you do decide to decorate the space:

---

1 From an article you can find here: huffingtonpost.co.uk/vanessa-olorenshaw/the-red-tent-movement_b_8091348.html

★ Use red fabric – this can be anything, for example red sheets, throws, or fabric. Some Red Tents gather things together from the community and have a Red Tent bag which is passed around the venues so that they don't have to source new decorations every time they meet or keep remembering to bring them!

I have a Red Tent box, which I always offer if any other woman wants to use it to decorate their space. There is a Tent entrance that I made myself, which I can hang up at the entrance door. So that's very beautiful. And then lots of material of red and orange and purple and pink. And it was lovely to think about all the stories these fabrics had absorbed over the years.
Susan

★ Welcome women with a sign on the door or create an entrance using material or cloth hanging from the ceiling or doorframe for women to enter through. We offer a welcome poster that you can download from the Red Tent Directory website.

★ Create a centrepiece in the middle of the area where you plan to hold your circle. This is sometimes called an altar. We don't mean to imply any specific religious significance, what we mean by this is a place where special things go, and those items are respected and left in place for the duration of the time together. So we will use *centrepiece* here. Perhaps you could think of it as a sacred space rather than a religious one. The centrepiece might include a candle, flowers as well as objects or images that relate to the vision you have for Red Tents and for community and honour the sacredness of that in your life. They may also reflect the seasons and any theme you might have for that month's Tent. Your centrepiece can also include cards, books and pictures that symbolise the Red Tent for you or you might have some of these available for people to browse during your time together.

★ Create comfy places to sit. Whatever venue you are using, you can invite women attending to bring something they find comfortable to sit on. A cushion or some kind of seat. These can also help to decorate the space and make the circle look attractive. Being mindful that comfy means different things for people who may need more support or space. Some Tents, for example, have optional chairs or pop up chairs for those that need them.

★ Consider how and if to use scent. If you choose to use a diffuser or burner to burn essential oils that bring a pleasant or calming scent to your space remember that not all oils are safe for those who may be pregnant and that scent may affect those with breathing issues. Some people have high sensitivity to scent for a number of reasons, those who have migraines, who are autistic, or after toxic chemical exposure or medical treatments such as chemotherapy. So asking people for consent at your Red Tent before you introduce scent or even naming the intention to use it in the invitation to your Red Tent is both a respectful and inclusive practice Some people may need a space to be completely scent and fragrance free. [2]

★ Many Red Tents burn herbs to clean and clear the space. Herbs have been used for this cleansing purpose in a variety of traditions through-out history. We know that many Tents use White Sage following – often very loosely – Native American traditions that they may know little about and have little or no engagement with. We have done this in the past without thinking. Many Native peoples name this as harmful appropriation of their spiritual practice. And so we invite you, if this is your practice, to reconsider it.

★ On the Red Tent Directory website we offer more resources to support you in creating a welcoming space.

2   Read more about this in a resource by Leah Lakshmi Piepzna-Samarasinha, "Fragrance Free and Scent Free Guidelines" at brownstargirl.org/fragrance-free-femme-of-colour-genius

Creating a Beautiful Space Online

Then Covid-19 descended, but undeterred, our team of now four love-ly Silva Guardians, made use of Zoom technology and have continued meeting monthly, holding "Sunday Silva Zoom Gatherings". It's still a safe (albeit virtual) space, where we women of a certain age can share our deepest wounds and the big hurdles we may have overcome and have yet to explore, as well as be recognised and rejoiced in our wisdom, strength and beauty.

Reana

Of course, you may not be able to decorate online space in the same way that you can a communal space or your living room! But you might think of decorating the space you are sitting in when you join the online tent. Perhaps you could hang some material behind you? You might invite others joining to do this also.

I found a red sheet that I draped across the sofa behind me and I had a wander around the garden and found some plants in flower to put next to some candles I'd popped on the 'centrepiece', which was actually a chair I'd manoeuvred within camera view so it could be seen by the participants on the call.

Steph

When thinking about how to run Red Tents online we think about how to create a different space to that we might have become used to creating online for business meetings or a casual chat with friends – especially during Covid-19. Some of this may be about the simple rituals you conduct before you open the space, which might be similar to what you would do if you were meeting in person. Take some time to connect to yourself and your intention before the Red Tent starts. Also think about how you can hold space in a way that is welcoming and allows people to feel comfortable and to connect more deeply to one another.

Welcoming

A woman said to me that I held the space energetically and then when I had gone, she could no longer hold the space in the same way, so women stopped coming. She said, "I cannot do it like you, so it is not working." I explained that there isn't a right way, I don't do anything special, I am just here, being open, being aware of how everyone is and allowing women to speak while others listen. Women can come and talk about what they want, there is no pressure. Some women don't want to share the first time. They say they are just here to listen, and that is fine. There is nothing to fix. We are coming together to be in this space, and it is a safe place.
Susana

This section is about welcome: how we welcome other women to Red Tents and how we also welcome ourselves. It's also about developing simple rituals around preparing for and opening your Red Tent space.

The word ritual may have lots of associations to you. When we speak about it in this chapter, we want to invite you to think about ritual as a practice or a sequence of practices that you can get familiar with and repeat. You can think of these as things you do that create space for the Red Tent in your life and therefore frame how you open up the space for others and invite them in. The rituals we discuss here are about honouring yourself, the space and the other women who come to it. We think about these rituals as being created with intention. As a result, they come alive in your life as well.

We want to invite you to think about the idea of having rituals as being about creating a sense of purpose and a sense of your Red Tent time and space as being different from the everyday flow of your life. When you show up and welcome people with this sense of creating an alternative kind of space clear in your mind, it's much easier to invite that energy in others too.

With the Red Tent, we are deliberately deciding not to create the kind of gathering we might create in many other parts of our lives. In this space we seek to welcome a more restful and nurturing space and to let go of our need to fix, judge and comment on everything other women say. We are intentionally allowing ourselves and one another to just be and feel whole in ourselves. For some people, this is something they rarely or never normally experience. This is why preparing yourself to host a Red Tent, whether it is in your own home, someone else's or in a public space is important. It's vital to take a few moments to sense the importance of what you are creating and remember why it matters to you.

Welcoming Yourself First

You might find that you rarely slow down. There are always things to do. Maybe you often find yourself speeding up to get things done so that at the end of it you can relax. But those moments seldom arrive. Carving out time and space to let the minutes pass gradually is a brave act and an important practice, and in our experience it can help us to show up in our lives – and Red Tents – feeling a little more grounded and whole.

And so to welcome yourself you may need to slow down, disengage from the need to be busy, embrace some quiet, hang up your roles for a few hours and just be yourself without all the trimmings of doing. We invite you to think about what kind of preparation rituals you might need in order to welcome this kind of space at your Red Tent.

REFLECTIVE QUESTIONS

★ What things help you to feel whole and nurtured?

★ What rituals would help you be open to create that kind of space?

★ How could you create some of this for yourself in the hours before your actual Red Tent?

Mads told us about how for her, the moment she starts preparing food for the Red Tent, she, "starts getting into that space". As she cooks her contribution to the shared refreshments, she feels that she starts to 'drop-in' to the Red Tent energy. You could say that this is her preparation ritual.

Your preparation might be very different. You might need some time alone or time out in nature. You might have other responsibilities that mean you have to rush on the day of the Red Tent, but perhaps you can find twenty minutes the day before that you can devote to something that helps you prepare. You might only have time to get a special piece of clothing or jewellery that for you evokes the Red Tent and spend a moment putting it on and sensing that the Red Tent is about to begin. Many Red Tents ask women to wear red as a way to unify those present. It is also about preparation for what is ahead, a bit like shedding one identity and putting on another. Whatever your own preparation ritual we invite you to create your own personal way of entering into the space before you begin. Something that helps you prepare and to show up to welcome other women.

Welcoming Others: Opening the Door

Women often bring a red scarf or wear something red. The red is connected to the blood of our ancestors. When we start a Red Tent we do a ceremony where each woman takes the red thread around their wrist and passes it around the circle so they feel connected together. As we do this, we think of our families and the connection with the women who have given birth to us and their mothers and grandmothers.

Susana

Welcoming women into a Red Tent space is important particularly if they have never entered this kind of gathering before. For many of us entering a new space where we may not know anyone can be really scary. As you welcome women to the Red Tent keep that in mind. Resist the temptation to hide yourself in comfortable familiar conversation with those you already know. Allow your welcome to the space to come from the heart and be genuine.

We've tried to ask for no small talk when people arrive because we want to keep it really clear and clean, then people know it is a different thing to their everyday. But then it's tricky for new people. So sometimes chatting is part of the welcoming and lets someone feel comfortable and arrive gradually.

Lily

For many women, the most difficult time can be the beginning, before the more structured part of the Red Tent starts. Be conscious of this and think about what might make your space feel nurturing and welcoming. It might be some gentle relaxing music, it could be that there are things to look at, perhaps books or pictures.

Don't underestimate the power of really paying attention to women as they arrive, seeing them as they enter the venue. Remember to give them basic information about what will happen at the Red Tent, where to put their coats, bags or shoes or any food they have chosen to contribute. This is a good time to check whether someone has any needs that you need to accommodate for them to feel welcome and able to participate. This may be having a chair to sit on, or asking their preferred language for those Red Tents which are multilingual.

For women who know each other already, this might be a time to catch up and chat. Make sure this *arrivals* part of the Tent is time-bound, so that your Red Tent doesn't become only a chatty kind of space. St. Albans Red Tent now has a woman designated as a *gatekeeper* at each of their Red Tent gatherings to help ensure that women are welcomed well and that the door is closed at a certain point. This is all communicated ahead of time in their invitation to their Red Tent.

Welcoming Guidelines

Introduce yourself and make new women welcome, but do not put pressure on them to engage physically or verbally on arrival. For many, especially those on the autism spectrum, being in a new space is sensorily overwhelming, and any additional demands to interact will be overloading and deeply stressful. For those communicating in a second language, again, this might be an overwhelming time.

If a woman seems like she doesn't want to engage or is looking stressed when she comes in, share with her where she can leave her coat, the location of the toilet (a necessary escape module for many during overwhelm), where refreshments are (drinking tea or water is a soothing and regulating activity) and if you have an area where the books are.

This gives the woman a brief orientation of the space and pointers of things to do that are not social whilst she acclimatises to the new space. A word on physical contact: whilst many of us may hug friends as a greeting and in some parts of the world greetings involve physical contact such as a kiss on the cheek, some women who come to your Red Tent may feel more comfortable with a no-contact greeting especially when you first meet them. Those with OCD, anxiety or on the autism spectrum may actively dislike physical contact with strangers, as may those with compromised immune systems. Be respectful, ask someone you are meeting for the first time, "Is it okay if I hug you?", rather than initiating what feels comfortable to you and don't be offended if the answer is "no".

Opening Ritual

We always have an altar where we reflect the moon cycles and the seasons. We have the ritual of lighting three candles. We always have a meditation. We sometimes sing, to get voices into the space first.
Laura and Lou

Once the women have arrived, and been welcomed into the space individually, it is time to gather as a group, to open the circle. Many women worry about this aspect of how to move into sacred space, how to start…

Firstly, find a way to get the attention of the women in the room, perhaps ring a bell, or turn off some of the main lights. Invite the women to sit in a circle.

Once everyone is seated, you might want to use a simple opening ritual. We share some examples from different Red Tents for inspiration but any simple way to mark the moment would work. Lighting candles on the centrepiece is a common way to do this.

A Simple Opening Ritual

We light this first candle to represent all the women who have come before us.

We light this second candle to honour ourselves, all those present, including those that are gathering at a Red Tent around the world at this time.

We light this third candle to symbolise the women who are yet to come into the world.

We evolved a tradition over months and months of doing the Red Tent. It finally got into something that was more of a format, but it always was open for change and suggestion.

To open the circle, we had a tray in the middle of the circle with little tea light candles on it, and we'd invite people to light their tea lights. We said, "This is the darkest time of the month and we're here to reflect each other's light. To gather around this warm hearth together."

We invited people to light their tea light, introduce themselves, and introduce their matrilineal line in whatever way they wanted, if it was biological or if it was naming their teachers: to name women who they descended from in some way. And then to call in someone. So, if there's a sister that you're thinking of that you want to invite into this circle who's not here, to call them in and then to send healing to someone or something. We'd go around and each woman would do that introduction and light her candle. And so, by the end, all the candles were lit.

That was our way of officially opening the circle. Then after that it really was just about whatever arises.

Emily

We would open the circle by lighting the three candles… And if there was something happening, particularly that felt pertinent at that time, I might bring that into the ritual, like, for example, those experiencing domestic violence during the coronavirus times. I would always do some breathing or mindfulness for a couple of minutes before we'd start talking, just so that people can actually feel present or it might even just be as simple as three breaths.

Lily

Our local Red Tent has now met twice online and have found, with conscious awareness on holding the sacred, it has really served in this time of virus. We still burn fragrant herbs (the holder lights the herbs and describes the smell or asks the women to recall it), sing a welcome song, and have found guided visualisation really helpful and supportive, as well, of course, as women being able to really speak about how the lockdown is for them. There's something about remembering to bring the body and her senses into the Tent – to ask women to feel into their bodies, their other senses.

Debbie

We developed a guide to hosting a Red Tent which we provided for each woman who was taking on this role. It gave a run through of how to welcome women into the space and provided an example of what to say. For example, include in your own words something on the lines of the following: "this is our time to leave all responsibilities aside, leave our caretaking of children, family and friends aside, leave our job persona aside, so that we can be fully present here just for ourselves. Many of us have wonderful skills in therapy, healing, counselling etc. but let's use this time to direct that inwards to ourselves, so that we keep this space free of our professional needs. This is our time to speak and be heard so that we can hear our own inner wisdom and be guided by it. This is a time to listen with open hearts without trying to fix each other or give advice." We invite those present to notice their own energy levels and emotions (vulnerable/tired, or upbeat/energetic etc.) and notice what they need for themselves to take care of and honour that energy during our time together.

Aisha

Creating Rituals for your Red Tent

There are many ways, beyond the practicalities of chairs and decorations, in which you can use ritual to support your Red Tent in a way that feels intentional, powerful and connective.

Many Red Tents have used practices from traditions other than their own or spiritual practices from another part of the world to help them to do this. In this book we want to invite you into a place of reflection and ask you to think about whether or not what you are currently doing is appropriate? In some cases, there may be someone from the lineage or culture where you are borrowing a tradition from present at your Tent. Sharing our traditions together in equitable and communal space is not something we think we should stop. In fact, let's do more of it!

What we do want to question is the appropriation of spiritual and cultural traditions without acknowledging or knowing their origins and using them as our own. That's appropriation and it's harmful.

I'm always amazed at a woman that will ship in white sage or palo santo to the UK and then recite a prayer for the four directions Native American style while banging on a drum from India.

As we can see right now with America burning, times need to change, understandings need to change. It is no longer acceptable to walk with a sage stick, in a bindi, singing African lullabies if you are of European heritage. Haven't the Europeans stolen enough from the Indigenous peoples of the Americas and Africa? There are clear Indigenous voices demanding this stops.

We need to find a way forward and reach for what is most appropriate and least likely to cause pain to others.

Nicola [3]

---

3   Nicola Goodall and her work can be found at Red Tent Doulas: redtentdoulas.co.uk

Cultural Appropriation

What is cultural appropriation and why should we think about it in relation to Red Tent spaces and rituals? Here's a definition from Maisha Z. Johnson: "Cultural appropriation is when somebody adopts aspects of a culture that's not their own. But that's only the most basic definition. A deeper understanding of cultural appropriation also refers to a particular power dynamic in which members of a dominant culture take elements from a culture of people who have been systematically oppressed by that dominant group."[4]

Why does it matter if we use practice and customs that originally come from somewhere else? Well, as Maisha says, power is an important element of this. All cultures are, in some way, both in flux and formed in relationship. But in the article, "What's Wrong with Cultural Appropriation? These 9 Answers Reveal Its Harm" – which we invite you to read for yourself – Maisha gives a number of compelling reasons why, when people from a dominant cultural or group 'borrow' from a group that has been oppressed, particularly through genocide, slavery or colonisation. Appropriation trivialises collective trauma, allows us to like and use cultural artefacts without questioning or dismantling injustice. It makes things that some groups may have been vilified for seem somehow appealing and 'cool' for those of a dominant group.

Land is spiritual. Land is not just a piece of property. It's much more than that. It's where we are born and where we bury the dead and where we get our food. So, to most Africans, land is really, really spiritual. And when people are separated from that which feeds them, they get hurt and fragmented, they're heartbroken. That's why there have been many wars about land issues, although sometimes people don't understand. They think that it's about material or acquiring material things, but it's more than that. It's about our ancestors, that's where they are, that's where they are buried. Can you imagine going into a place where someone else's ancestors are buried and you make it your own and you forget that they

---

4   Find Maisha Johnson's article "What's Wrong with Cultural Appropriation? These 9 Answers Reveal its Harm" at everydayfeminism.com/2015/06/cultural-appropriation-wrong

might haunt you.

Hope Chigudu[5]

So for example, when we 'borrow' a Native American ritual, such as using the burning of white sage in a specific way, called *smudging*, we are taking for ourselves a spiritual practice from a people whose land has been colonised, whose rituals have been banned and who are still marginalised and oppressed in contemporary life. We are stealing a ritual for which Native Americans have been oppressed and punished. When we do so, it's as if we are erasing a culture and their traditions and ignoring their persecution. It is like we are taking a tiny part of that ritual and sanitising it in our hands. While we may benefit by appearing more interesting, spiritual or quirky we will not face harm or be ostracised.

If we are raced as white we can do so comfortably and without consequence is because we are afforded more power and privilege within the system of colonisation and white supremacy. When we do this without defending the rights of Native people to have their land and lives decolonised we are also borrowing from a culture without standing in solidarity with the people who have suffered for it.

That is not to say that traditions of burning herbs in ritual space do not exist in other cultures. They do. But we also don't think that simply stopping burning sage and appropriating another practice is a solution for this. Sophie Macklin reflects this when she says, "I think what people have tried to do with the awareness of cultural appropriation and say, smudging, they're like, 'Oh we don't smudge, we're Saining, which is Scottish.' And they are saying this is from my lineage…and still not holding it in its cultural context with the depth of understanding of what Saining actually is in that Scottish tradition. And so I think one of the first things is that we need to slow down a bit and acknowledge the depth of loss and alienation that we are coming from and that there's not an easy answer in lineage because it very quickly falls apart unless you are going to start going down a (racial) purity line."[6]

When we assume that because we have a relative from a specific part of the

5   Hope Chigudu in conversation with Mary Ann Clements, Healing Solidarity 2020 conference, Welcoming Change. Recordings available via healingsolidarity.org

6   Sophie Macklin instagram.com/sophieamacklin

world that gives us the automatic right to take its cultures and traditions as our own, we may affectively be appropriating from our ancestors' cultures. Making the assumption, as Sophie says that "I have this lineage therefore I have a right to possess this" is dangerous. It not only commodifies cultures and traditions making an assumption that they are static but also risks aligning us with the racial purity assumed by far-right groups and fascist movements.

She continues, "The ethno-nationalist movement is growing dangerously and it's important to be working against that." One way in which we can do that is question our right to possess practices and assume them as our own even if they come from places where some of our ancestors came from.

When Black and Indigenous communities assert their right to ancestral practices they are questioning power and reclaiming what white supremacy has stolen and erased. It is completely different when white nationalists assert ancestral lineage and reassert racial difference and supremacy and perpetuate dangerous divisions in our world. They infer that they have a right to do this, because they are white. We invite you to tread carefully therefore, particularly if you are white and exploring ancestral practices. Explore and connect with your ancestors and their traditions by all means, but always question the extent to which you might be inadvertently appropriating from the past and aligning yourself with a nationalist sentiment or concepts of racial purity. We need to resist these in as many ways as we can in our world at this time.

Remember also that we each have a huge number of ancestors. If we go back nine generations, we each have up to 2,048 great-grandparents[7], and if we go far enough back, we probably share one with one another and with you!

When thinking about cultural appropriation, we invite you to understand that white supremacy and patriarchal capitalism have violently erased many facets of culture over generations and so the hunger for practices and rituals to call our own is real. At the same time if we borrow from other cultures and traditions, without any understanding or knowledge of what we are doing and in turn profit from doing so or call it our own, we are participating in the continued commodification, erasure, and colonisation of Indigenous practices. We can easily become part of the problem.

We know this is a difficult and complex topic. We invite you to bring the questions into your Red Tent space knowing that there are no simple answers. There's no 'right way' to do it. There's no simple fix. We are writing at a time

---

7   We saw this in an Instagram post originally shared by @lyricalzen on Ancestral Mathematics.

when these questions are beginning to be asked more widely in online spaces and conversations and it's tempting to want to be the person who doesn't slip up or make a mistake. Particularly as white women we know the temptation to want to make sure that we are 'one of the good ones' in contrast to others. [8] We might even say to ourselves that other Tents are doing things wrong, but we are in the right. We might want to judge examples of appropriation we deem to be harmful while justifying our own. Sometimes it is easier to point the finger than to unpack our own assumptions and what supports them.

I believe my part in taking rituals from Indigenous traditions stems from my own hunger for what is absent in my own lineage. The traditions in my family come from Roman Catholicism and lacked any nature-based practices. Many people in my family have grown vegetables, flowers and herbs for pots, pans and vases but not for ceremony. As someone who gravitates towards the outdoors whenever possible, finding rituals from Indigenous cultures that had a reverence and deep connection with the natural world was consistent with what I valued. I greedily took them as my own treasures. My privilege both gave me the sense of entitlement to cherry pick from traditions and made me impervious to the harm I was complicit in.
Aisha

We invite you to reach for a healthier balance collectively within your Red Tent between an awareness that we all have many ancestors and an understanding of the function of white supremacy and colonisation in our world today and in particular over the last five hundred years.

Some of our ancestors may have profited from silence, from slavery, from the erasure and oppression of Indigenous peoples and customs. Some of them may have lost things, been oppressed, been vilified and harmed.

When we understand that white supremacy, patriarchy, capitalism and colonisation in our world have such a huge impact, then we can commit to trying to take steps to liberate ourselves from them. And we can't do that by stealing a practice from here and there and colonising it for ourselves.

8   Mary Ann discusses this idea further in her article here medium.com/@ maryannmhina/what-capacities-might-we-as-white-people-in-international-development-need-to-build-in-ourselves-49e765a3151b

We invite you to ask these questions, not just for yourself in private, but in community, in your Red Tent.

If you have learnt practices, teachings or traditions from other parts of the world, ask yourself, who have you learnt them from? And who is profiting?

How might you invite accountability and repair for custom and traditions you have benefited from inequitably in the past?

Is there a way that you can support communities without making a fuss but perhaps by making a financial donation?

What ways might you find to begin to repair and make reparations knowing that it is again not something you can quickly fix and tick off as 'done' but rather may well be the process of a lifetime?

For me there was relief in naming it. Naming the feeling inside, the unease, the awkwardness as I practiced a cultural practice that I was not connected to, knowledgeable about or in active solidarity with... But something clicked and I was shocked I hadn't seen it before. It was so clear. I cannot own a sacred practice. I cannot assume connection when it is not reciprocated. I cannot take what I want without seeing what has been lost. I have not suffered the cost to preserve a practice when it faced erasure. I am me, not someone else from somewhere else. They are not my stories, my prayers or my personal struggles. It explained moments I hadn't fully understood and shifted the lens.

I felt a sense of urgency to fix something intangibly wrong. But this was a big piece I realised. And rushing to do something, anything, was part of the same colonial mindset which had made me presume it was okay in the first place. I needed to sit with the scale of oppression that I was ingrained in and ask how I was perpetuating it. I wanted to reflect on how I could stop causing harm, stop making assumptions, literally just stop and listen. I knew more than anything that this was about seeing the larger context and not getting lost in my own drama. So for me, it's part of a long spiral of unlearning, feeling into the corners of my disconnection and grief. There is emptiness and it wants to be filled but I have also realised that it needs to be felt.

Aisha

Capitalism loves to package stuff up and sell it. It loves to make a commodity of the healing practices that were shared in sacred ways in communities. White supremacy loves to take the benefits without honouring or rewarding the lineage. It loves to tell you that, as a white person, you have every right to take what others have shared with you and own it as yours. It's called colonisation and doesn't just apply to land, but also to thoughts, traditions, objects and ideas. All of these systems are built on the idea of extraction, of profit and of most of us being oppressed for the benefit of the few. Patriarchy also loves to tell you that as a woman in all of this, it's your fault and you must fix it.

Within the context of the world as it is right now, the answers to these questions are complex and what we need to do, we think, is find ways, in community, to bring our awareness to the questions rather than jumping to any quick-fix answer. We need to learn to sit – in circle – with the discomfort of it all.

I always felt a dis-ease when I encountered practices that seemed dissociated from their spiritual lineage within Red Tents and other women's spaces. I couldn't voice it for a long time or name it. But I felt dis-ease. And I couldn't bring myself to promote or use practices that felt this way to me.

I think there was a part of me that understood some of what we are exploring in this chapter instinctively but for some time, many years actually, I couldn't put words to it and perhaps that was in a way white supremacy active through me preventing me from taking the risk of speaking up. I just felt funny about it, but also knew that I had found a sense of community in Red Tent spaces in other ways and so I was left with this internal conflict and always the question: Is there something wrong with me that I don't quite 'get it'? Am I in some way not spiritual enough?

Now I think this discomfort was really a sense of some knowing that I couldn't quite consciously express that some things really didn't feel okay to me because they were appropriative and it has been freeing to realise this. It has also enabled me to get out of the place of quiet complicity – which is just as harmful as promotion – and speak.

Mary Ann

REFLECTIVE QUESTIONS

We invite you to start by considering honouring the traditions and rituals that have been taught to you personally by your own family and community. This can be done as a group also, grieving the loss of ritual as a Red Tent circle together. A lot of what we are inviting here is for you to sit with these challenging questions without jumping to easy solutions or answers and so we invite you to consider collectively making space for this exploration. Perhaps you could create your own rituals to explore grief more fully together.[9]

★ What were the rituals around you as you grew up?

★ How was the sacred honoured in the daily life of your family and community? If the answer is that it wasn't, you might want and need to acknowledge that loss.

★ How can you bring a flavour of who you are and where you came from into a Red Tent space?

★ How can you honour the different lineages of the women who attend your Red Tent? Remember that people of many different lineages and cultures may attend your Tent. Invite people to share from their lineages in appropriate ways that honour them. Share traditions in ways that feel just and equitable.

★ How might you choose together to create your own simple rituals? Remembering always to honour anything that has influenced or inspired them.

---

9   Try this podcast for some ideas: changemakingwomen.com/57-practicing-collective-grief-with-sophie-macklin

Suggestions for Clearing Space

Remember that a solution to cultural appropriation is not necessarily assuming that you can use a practice because you have read on the internet that it may have been used by your distant ancestors.

I have some Mexican heritage but grew up knowing this only as a story without any traditions or rituals associated with it. I simply knew that my grandmother's name was from Mexico. I know a bit more now and I believe I do have some heritage from that part of the world. However, none of its rituals and practices were passed down to me and it is also a place with its own history of colonisation and appropriation. If I was to now choose to look up 'space clearing rituals from Mexico' on the internet and assume I can possess and use them as my own, because I have an ancestor who moved to this island from there in the nineteenth century, I would be missing the point. We don't have an automatic right to possess and appropriate our ancestors' rituals in this way. They are part of the fabric of life and communities that have, in many cases, been decimated by colonisation. Calling in liberation means asking difficult questions and feeling together – as a Red Tent community – towards practices that we can call our own.

Mary Ann

This doesn't mean we can't explore our own ways to clear and cleanse space. Below we explore some ideas for foundation of methods that you might use to prepare a space or provide a cleansing ritual for those entering it which draw on the elements in our natural world – as many different communities have done throughout human history. Our invitation is to explore what feels congruent and useful as a spiritual practice for you and your own Red Tent community.

All our food comes from nature. We breathe, air comes from nature, water comes from nature, our being comes from nature. Who told us to disconnect from nature? How did this happen? … Connect with nature, with its healing powers. Connect with nature and appreciate what nature does for us.

Connect with nature in a way that reminds us that if we destroy this, we are finished.

Hope Chigudu [10]

Water

To bring in the water element, collect water from a local source to where you live, anything from a spring, river, stream, sea, tap or rainwater to use as part of your ritual. Once you have your water then either leave it as it is or add petals or herbs grown locally. Or add purifying properties to the water such as sustainably sourced charcoal, salt or slices of lemon.

Decide how you want to move it around the room either with a steam infuser, a cluster of ice, a spray bottle to create droplets in the space or a little blessing bowl for self-anointing or handwashing at the entrance.

If you want to provide a way for women to transition into the space, you could provide the water you have prepared along with handmade bath salts or natural soap from oils, herbs or petals. Invite each woman to wash her hands with intention and care before entering the space.

Fire

If you are holding a Red Tent outside you can have a fire, or bring it inside if you have a wood burner or equivalent. Fire is able to transform one element into another or release properties in scent or smoke. You might want to burn herbs or resin if it is rooted in your tradition and locally sourced. Many spiritual practices around the world use herbs in a variety of different ways. You might choose to take time to explore the herbs that grow abundantly where you are and are either native or at least well-established. Experiment with burning different plants but be sure to check for safety before you do this.

Lighting candles or an oil lamp and moving around the space is a potent metaphor. You could use candles that are special for a number of reasons: they are homemade or made in community, they are scented or decorated, they hold the passage of time by being used at multiple Tents. One Red Tent listed in the Directory carved the name of every woman who has ever attended on the candle. You could make oil lamps using locally sourced oil such as rapeseed, olive or sunflower oil.

If you want to welcome women in with fire they can be passed a light as

10 Hope Chigudu in conversation with Mary Ann Clements, Healing Solidarity 2020 conference, Welcoming Change. Recordings available via healingsolidarity.org

they come in or they could write down something they are letting go of in order to be present here and place it in the fire to burn.

Air

To bring in the air element you might want to use song or spoken word to prepare a space with intention. You can open the window if it is windy and welcome in some fresh air to literally clear the air. You can use breathing as a way to settle into a space and gradually relax.

If you want to bring in a symbolic aspect of air you can use feathers gleaned from the ground, so you know where they are from rather than buying them without knowledge of how they are sourced.

Earth

To bring in the earth element you can bring stones in the space. If you currently use crystals, look into how they are sourced as the majority of precious gems and minerals are extracted using child labour in dangerous and harmful settings,[11] not to mention the environmental impact of mining. Alternatively gather rocks that are part of your natural habitat: ones that you have collected for their shape and texture, ones that have markings of animals long deceased, ones that have shiny clusters of other rocks showing.

You might want to interpret earth as the abundance of seeds, plants, herbs, flowers, and fruits that are grown from the earth. Remember to cultivate anything you find in nature with respect and only take a little so the plant can continue to flourish. You might want to gather berries or make things to taste and share. Alternatively, you might want to bring in the soil from outside or invite each woman to bring a little from somewhere special to them like their garden or a local park.

If you want to bring women into the space with a ritual, you might use seeds or bulbs and invite them to write down something they want to grow in themselves metaphorically and then plant them together. Or you could ask each person to write on a stone something they are grateful for that they have in their life.[12]

---

11 theguardian.com/lifeandstyle/2019/sep/17/healing-crystals-wellness-mining-madagascar

12 We would like to extend our thanks to Mint Faery for sharing different ideas that she uses to clear space without appropriating other cultures youtube.com/watch?v=OmVIpEZ0-Ys&t=294s

It is about creating your own practice that is meaningful to you and your community.

We have a huge tradition of plant medicine here. We have protective herbs. And I'm starting to explore our understanding of tree medicine recently as it's not a part of our botanica I've ever really delved into before. Chat with your grandmothers, go to your national libraries and archives, read your old books.

Engage with the fact your medicine has been erased and fight to reinstate it. It's a matter of reclamation and it's super important. Encouraging women to do this has given me the great pleasure of watching countless women exploring their ancestral roots and connecting with their ancestors. It has been profound. It has been beautiful. They walk into their power.

Nicola

Emergent Ritual

We did use sage in Toronto but I'm starting a Red Tent [in California] and I don't think I'm going to do any of that. I don't feel comfortable with using Native American traditions in that way now, nor with the kind of circle where everyone says 'Aho!', because there's this awareness. Part of the Red Tents is about having words that we can own, and organic, emergent vocabulary and ritual and a sense that 'this is coming from us because it's not really from any time'. I mean, yes, there are quasi Biblical origins in the Red Tent, but I think it really is about a space where we can feel empowered to create our own, without having to be ashamed about it. I'd say it's emergent ritual. It's like something that comes from us that's always been in us. And so, it's important to use vocabulary that's ours, that comes from the circle.

Emily

We want to invite you to think about sharing practices at your Red Tent that have been brought and shared by a woman within the circle perhaps from her own traditions and daily life. To think of rituals and practices as something that everyone has access to is a powerful way to reflect on what Emergent Ritual might look like for each of us. And this only becomes possible if we are cognisant of the importance of paying attention to cultural appropriation and to what it means to seek to be in a more equitable relationship to one another, not just individually, but culturally as well.

If someone within a Red Tent offers an idea that connects them to their family, community or heritage traditions, then this can be welcomed into the space or those present can create something that feels significant to them in that moment.

We always ask at the beginning of our Tent if anyone has a tradition that they've been using that they feel would be appropriate here that they want to share. I remember one woman once she led a womb blessing that she had been taught somewhere, but she had never done anything like that with a group. She had some language that she spoke and then each person said that phrase to the next person and put their hand on their belly and a hand on their heart. We went around the circle and each person did it: people were in tears, it was really moving – it was the first time that this woman had led any kind of a group healing.
Emily

We invite you to simplify. To let go of the need to have the best ritual, the right tradition, the most spiritual thing. As we have already said, it may be more appropriate to grieve the loss, either by simply creating a grieving ritual around the letting go of practices you no longer want to use or grieving more generally the lack of practices to support us in our lives. Always remember that tradition is never static. There is not one ideal place for us to go back to in our practice. Cultures and their traditions and rituals are actually always in flux.

It's something that's triggered me in other women's circles when people act like: this is passed down from my sacred lineage. It's like, 'from where?' I've found that that sort of intense spirituality in terms of 'here's the way we do it' to be a barrier, a barrier to my safety to feeling connected to it and feeling like I can really own it. So one of my criteria in starting this Red Tent was that it was about lowering those barriers to access, really just allowing it to be pure and simple feminine energy space to connect, nurture, rest, slow down, just about honouring the wisdom that's in all of us and creating a space that can emerge in an organic way.

I think because of that, there were so many people who came, who hadn't done any sort of sacred feminine work at all and that they were able to feel safe and included and welcome and felt safe to speak. I know that there are a lot of women who have really studied and really, you know, feel that they're part of a lineage and that's awesome. But for me, I think that in the Red Tents that I'm a part of, I want everyone to feel safe and comfortable. So, it was very kind of grassroots, just whatever emerges, emerges and I think that that's really empowering, when people are invited to co-create and to acknowledge their own wisdom.

Emily

Weaving Change

The answers to how we might build culture and avoid appropriation are not always simple and we may not always 'get it right'. As Kenneth Jones and Tema Okun have suggested, the very desire for perfectionism may also, to some extent, have its roots in the emergence of whiteness and white supremacy. [13] Allow yourself to muddle through, get it wrong and apologise and correct things. Allow yourself to be learning and acknowledging and changing things when it feels right. The challenges and questions you come across are something that can be brought to the circle for exploration and discussion also as part of your Red Tent.

We have changed our own practices over time and built our awareness. Part of this journey has also been about reflecting on the traditions and lineages that we do feel connected to. Strengthening our connection to those helps us to love and appreciate the diversity of others. That feels, to us, very different to needing to borrow or appropriate because we feel we don't have practices that we can own or that have emerged from us.

Running a Red Tent as an act of resistance in a supremacist system that

---

13 Jones, Kenneth and Okun, Tema. *Dismantling Racism: A Workbook for Social Change Groups*

has colonised and raced us is not simple, but we invite you to feel into these questions and explore your own answers to developing practices that are emergent and authentic for you and those you share your Red Tent space with. We invite you to think this through for yourself and find what works for you. Don't be afraid to experiment and make mistakes.

We don't need to appropriate other people's cultures to challenge systems of oppression. You can start simply. Day to day. By rejecting their hold.

There has to be a way to live in more equitable and just relationship to one another, to honour one another's traditions and influences and to advocate for justice together.

Let's move towards that.

REFLECTIVE QUESTIONS

★ How will you welcome people to your Red Tent?

★ What ritual or practice will you use to open the space?

★ Reflect for yourself on your tradition and lineage. How can aspects of what is important to you be offered to a Red Tent?

★ How might you invite people to bring their own traditions, rituals, stories and ideas and contribute them to a co-sourced gathering?

★ How could this deepen your connection to each other and what might it lead to in terms of our rich viewpoint of culture, heritage and history?

★ All of this applies just as much online as in person and so if you are holding your Tent online how will you honour your lineage and enable people to bring what they want to of their traditions too?

★ What will you do if someone brings into Red Tent a ritual that others in the circle find inappropriate? Perhaps because of its religious significance or meaning for them or they sense that it is appropriated? How will you explore and resolve any conflict about this?

★ And how will you enable women who want to choose for themselves and opt out of anything they might not feel comfortable participating in for any reason?

Beginning the Circle

We generally talk about our agreements, how are we showing up here? To make sure that it was a really brave and safe space. We want it to make all of that explicit too. So, we just offer the circle to say, "What will make you feel safe and comfortable to show up as fully as you can over the next two hours?" And confidentiality, we usually talk about that, and that it's not a space for problem-solving. It's about just witnessing and holding space.

Emily

We have very clear guidelines. Everybody knows what they are. I'm not always a person who likes those structures, but actually, it really does help. All of these rules are to allow us to be able to relax so that the women can do just that.

So, we ask people to meet and chat and have tea downstairs. And then, at two o'clock, we go upstairs to the sacred space. We ask people in the invitation to commit to the four hours in advance. And we asked them to please stay for the whole time, so that we can share the space. We have a break roughly halfway through, after we've done the sharing. And then we have a shared dinner afterwards at six if they want to stay, and a lot of people do.

Lou

I think that writing down everything was really helpful so that we weren't saying "We hold all the knowledge." Instead, we're saying, "Here is some guidance. If you're going to host, then read this." Every single person received that same support. And we would sit together in the steering circle, and I just would think, "Wow, seriously? You're questioning everything?" I'd just come from the city where things are really, "Do this, do that, get it

done." And you're discussing how to introduce the Red Tent when women arrive, and how it's going to be received and do we want to use this word or that? So when I went into the Red Tent and I just thought, "Ah, I see now why it was important," and my whole heart opened, my whole self just had a space to be…and not just be but feel held by the structure, because we had so beautifully considered everything in detail beforehand.
Elaine

As we discussed earlier, it is helpful if you share at the outset how the Red Tent time will be structured and to be clear about what shared agreements you do or don't have for the space. Common agreements include:

★ No advice, fixing or responding unless requested.

★ Not talking when others are speaking.

★ Holding confidentially and refraining from gossiping or repeating or commenting on what we hear in a Red Tent: "What is said in circle stays in circle."

★ Ensuring everyone present has the opportunity to speak.

★ No promotion of our services, offerings or businesses within the Red Tent space.

★ Don't share from a place of trying to point out that your own issues, challenges or wounds are somehow worse or superior to those of someone else. Stay conscious of how oppression can operate in this space. How we can react to one another, feel superior or lesser to one another, use our feelings in ways that burden or attack one another and try to stay in what is yours, in what is really true for you.

★ Try to listen and share from a place of personal reflection and honesty rather than debate or discussion.

★ Respect the time agreements for sharing.

★ If you are online be clear how you will decide who goes next. We tend to prefer being intuitive about this, but some people do a virtual passing on of the space to speak. For us this brings up all kinds of questions about "Why didn't anyone want to pass to me?" which we think can be unhelpful and risk triggering things for people, and so when we meet virtually, we prefer to leave it to women to indicate when they are ready to speak.

In the rest of this book, you'll read many examples of how different Red Tents spend their time together. What is important is being clear from the outset what your plans for the Red Tent are. It's also okay if those plans have an element of flexibility. We often start a Red Tent simply knowing that we will hold a circle at the beginning and end, facilitating check-in and check-out, but not quite knowing what activities we might do in the middle.

This is one of the things that makes Red Tents different from a workshop for us: we don't need to have every detail prepared. We just want to have some shared agreements and a structure where we say: we will eat together, we will take breaks, we will share where we are at and do some restful and nurturing things together. Exactly what those are might evolve from members of the group as the Red Tent unfolds. This is part of the letting go which we invite you to think about and hold as an intention in relation to your Red Tent. You don't have to know it all, you just need to commit to holding space and creating the opportunity for women to meet in this way and at the same time having a simple structure you can share with everyone present can help them feel comfortable in the space you are creating.

Sitting in a circle and holding space in this way can be a daunting experience the first few times you do it. Even if you have led groups before, holding a circle takes us out of our familiar conditions and asks us to focus on being connected to the circle we are holding, rather than leading it in a way we might be accustomed to in other parts of our lives.

I was nervous about introducing the idea of sitting in circle to women who had never come across this before, as I was unsure of how it might be received. But after the first few slightly awkward sharings, we have all become more trusting in this – seeing for ourselves how it has benefitted each of us – how little pressure there is for anyone to go further with sharing than they are comfortable, and knowing you're allowed to share just as deeply as you wish. Understanding that tears are allowed to flow if they come, you don't need to dab them up, and that anything we say is not judged but held as both valid and confidential. It's proved to be a real joy to all of us and has brought both sisterhood within the circle and friendship in everyday life between women who may not otherwise know one another.

Lara

Check-in

The women come and we close the doors, so if women come late, they don't enter. And then we burn herbs and guide a visualisation or meditation helping us to be in our body, be connected to the earth, to the moon. I like to call all the women in my family or the women with whom I feel connected. We invite the women of the circle to speak their name. So we have a time where we hear the names of all these women around us and then we start the circle, asking each to share why they're here and how they are.

Camille

For us, a central part of what makes a gathering a Red Tent is a sharing circle that all women in attendance take part in. This is often called a *check-in* circle. This is the moment you share your name with the group and tell them about what is going on for you. Rather than checking into a hotel, think of it more like checking inside a pocket that holds all your feelings and thoughts that maybe don't always see the light of day or get spoken or heard. This usually opens the main part of the Red Tent once everyone has arrived and is the space in which women are invited to share what is going on for them, to speak honestly and be witnessed by the rest of the women in the circle. Having time and quiet to talk about yourself in a personal way can be a big deal, especially the first few times you do it. Being invited to take some time for yourself and talk about how you feel in this moment of your life, right now, is in itself a gift. But also something many of us fear because it is so seldom invited or accepted.

Talking Objects

A good way to facilitate check-ins from each woman in the circle is using a talking object. We want to acknowledge that talking sticks have been used historically by many native peoples including Aboriginal groups in Australasia, Native American tribes on the American continent and different groups living on the African continent as well. The use of talking pieces in Red Tent spaces likely originates from North America where the use of talking sticks by healing traditions has appropriated Native customs, often without honouring, naming or supporting them.

What feels important to us in this particular case is that we honour the many traditions from which we draw, knowing that we don't know everything about them. So we introduce the idea of a talking object here, acknowledging all of the peoples that have come before us that have used talking pieces to discuss, witness, honour, share and make peace with one another and also being clear that our suggestions here come from our own practice which may not mirror any of those traditions. The idea we have of this is that a stone, stick or other object is passed from one person to the next. When they are holding the object, it is their turn to speak. They may also pass the object on if they are not ready to speak. This way of indicating who is speaking helps to create the flow and intention of the circle, ensures that everyone has an opportunity to share and prevents the circle from developing into a conversation or advice-giving session, as each person has their own opportunity to speak and be heard when they have the object. When they have finished, the focus moves as they pass it on often in a clockwise direction. Think of it like the winding up of a clock. Later at the end of a circle the direction can reverse to symbolise unwinding the space you have created.

It's important to be clear about timing in these check-in rounds. For example, to make clear whether each woman will have two, five or ten minutes to speak, depending on how much time you have and how many women are present. Once this is made clear it is important to have a way of holding women to this as a collective shared agreement. This means that someone needs to time each check-in and there needs to be an agreed symbol for alerting women when their time is up.

I would invite people to speak from the heart in a way that is kind of spontaneous. Then we'd use the clock for timing how long we each got to speak, with the person who has just spoken doing the timing for the next person. Sometimes people are so engrossed in what the other person is saying that they totally forget to look at the clock. But usually it works out fine, and I have found that's quite a good strategy for timing – passing the clock along.
Lily

We always provided some suggestions of what to say to introduce the way that we transitioned into the held circle after the welcome part. We highlighted that everyone has a chance to share, but they can pass if they don't want to speak or need more time before speaking. We reminded them that this is a space to be heard, and to honour each other with our listening. We invited them to check in with their name and how they are feeling right now. Then we suggested that they can then ask those present to share the essence of what is going on in their life: "Whatever you want to express to feel present in this circle." In a large group, we suggested up to two minutes each and timed them. Letting them know that you would raise a hand to indicate when their time was up, but that they were encouraged to finish their sentence. Or in a big group we would simply introduce our names and say a few words and then split into smaller groups to have a longer time for sharing.
Aisha

If people speak longer than the time you've introduced, then they may need to be gently reminded that it is time for them to stop. It might be that you do so by acknowledging that there is perhaps a desire to have a longer time for sharing so after the check-in you could see if some or all of the group want to break into smaller groups for a longer round or deeper check-ins.

Another shared agreement is to invite everyone to speak from the place of 'I' and their own experience. A check-in is not a chance to resolve issues with someone else in the room. It is a place to share our own experience. It isn't a space to respond to what others have shared, and so it is good to be clear and have an agreement relating to that. That doesn't mean that difficult things won't come up. We provide some approaches to dealing with 'difficult things' that may come up in your circle later, as creating spaces where people feel able to be honest and bring their whole selves can often bring challenges. When people do bring up uncomfortable conversations it may actually be a sign that people feel able to share very openly but it might be also indicate that an earlier agreement was not sufficient and may need strengthening.

Ultimately, if there is something in a check-in that is clearly an attack on someone else or is racist or abusive there are times when you may have to stop a circle and intervene or to ask that something is 'parked' on one side until it can be dealt with in another way.

How to decide when to intervene

★ If you sense in your belly that something that has been said is not acceptable and has caused harm within the circle, stop the circle. Ask for a moment. Take a breath. Then, if it feels possible, voice your concern clearly, using what the person actually said, so: "When you said (whatever they said) I felt that it was (describe the problem) and I would like us to (take a break/discuss this together/ park this issue and discuss it later with those concerned)"

★ If you do need to intervene in this way remember that you are breaking the agreements of the circle space. Know that you are doing that for a deliberate reason and your wish is to maintain as much safety as possible in the space.

★ Try to do this in a shame-free way, owning your own judgements as "I felt/judged it was problematic" rather than "You were prob- lematic" and giving others the chance to correct you if you have facts wrong.

Be aware that if you are intervening about something that has been said that applies to a specific person or people in the group, rather than a generally offensive or unacceptable comment, you may wish to seek their input and at the same time this may be a burden for them.

Creating a Brave Space

The simplicity of the women's circle setting is attractive. There are few ex-pectations, in my experience, other than showing up, being respectful, and perhaps bringing an offering or gift and something to be eaten or drunk together. Yet the potential rewards of sharing lives, vulnerabilities and experiences are great. Women's experiences are not the same, and there are often differing views amongst women. But in these interweaving stories, there are moments of humanity, emotion, empathy, connection and a lack of judgement, advice or derision that is so refreshing.
Madeleine

In a circle everyone gets a chance to speak and be heard, and the rest of us do not get a right to reply. The only exception, as we explored above, is if you are intervening because you believe something someone has said is causing harm within the circle. This means that you, too, get to speak and share, and ask for support from the other women if you need it, knowing that they will only offer support or advice if it is directly requested.

This is a chance, unusual for most of us, to share without anyone trying to fix us, answer us, make things better or give us advice. In our experience there is immense power in this. It helps to democratise the space and levels out all our many differences into an appreciation of our common humanity as women. It both sets the foundation for community and strips away the need to present the shiniest version of ourselves or the most broken parts to be fixed.

I remember it being a totally different way of interacting than I'd ever been used to before. No one really talked about their personal lives or relationships or work, everything was very anonymous. It was years before I really knew what anyone did or if they had a partner, you know, like sometimes people would disclose stuff, but it was stripped back to how they were experiencing things rather than the detail of their lives.
Lily

We can take off the roles of rescuing each other and hushing the words spoken with an answer. The rawness of our words can flow from our mouths and linger in the air fully formed and invited to stay. Perhaps we so often feel that we need to respond and give advice because that is generally the way many of us have been conditioned. In our patriarchal culture we sense offering advice is part of what makes us feel useful and valued. Though our views and opinions may be marginalised in general, we can offer direction and guidance to our sisters. So this can feel uncomfortable at first.

We say: "If you want to be respected and honoured and the integrity held for you, please hold it for another." Any intention can be listened to. We're all equal here. There's no religion or politics that will stop me from listening to somebody, however uncomfortable that might be.
Susan

A basic expectation is that when one woman is sharing, she is not interrupted. Advice is not given without request. And what a woman talks about is not brought up again, unless invited by her. We experience that when women come together, we can be intuitive with each other without responding to what is said: we get what we need just by speaking and being heard. Our experience is that developing the art of listening to hear – rather than listening to give your input – can be transformational, both for the listener and the woman who is being listened to. This way of sitting together in a circle enables each woman to introduce herself and share how she is feeling. It also establishes a way of relating to each other that is valuable for the whole of the Red Tent.

I am so grateful to have witnessed so much: so many stories, feelings, experiences, including my own. We all have something to share, we all have times of feeling the need to be held, seen, nurtured and witnessed. I have learnt not to fix, over-mother or heal. But to trust in the process of being present, being here now, knowing that unconditional love is the only way.
Angie

Women's voices have often been silenced throughout history. Our voices have been dismissed as unreliable or unremarkable. This continues to the present day, as women who choose to speak out are shut down. The power of listening to a woman is healing. It gives her permission to vocalise her thoughts and experiences. It allows her the space to articulate what is important to her. By not responding we also give her permission to fully own all her thoughts and feelings. And it helps heal all the times we have been shut down or criticised or ridiculed for sharing our thoughts. Listening is an important tool to redress the imbalance.

It's also the case that some women's voices have been silenced by other women. That white feminism has often silenced the voices of Black women and of other women of colour. Queer and trans women's voices have been silenced too, as have those of gender-nonconforming people. Whilst listening to one another alone won't overcome this, listening deeply can be a powerful practice that chooses not to recreate this oppression.

In a challenging environment and society we create a new paradigm first by gathering together in the essence of solidarity and creativity, then bringing it out to the world to break taboos and change perceptions. We must start somewhere and we need the support of everyone.
Louise

Opening the Tent by inviting each woman to speak in this way is the glue that holds everyone together and builds connection. So, make sure that you do it with intention. Hold your intentions for yourself and consider also sharing these with the group of women sitting in circle with you. Remind women why they have come together. And then make sure that you speak to both confidentiality and the agreed finish time each time you meet so that everyone is clear. You might say something like:

Holding space in this way means allowing us to come as we are. Whether you are feeling joyous or irritated, closed or open…however you are in this moment. Each woman is welcomed exactly as she is. As we go around there will be an object passed to you. This is a talking piece. Everyone gets the opportunity to speak, if they wish. Take your time and say what you need to, ask for what you need or tell us what you would like to share. If you aren't ready to speak, then the talking piece will come back to you when and if you are ready. When a woman has the talking piece it is her space, so we don't respond with words, advice, or try to fix her tears or emotion. We listen, as best we can, to her sharing. Once she has finished the talking piece is then passed on.

Mads

Confidentiality means not mentioning anything a woman has shared outside of the circle itself – even later in the gathering – unless the woman herself initiates a conversation.

As Mary Ann helps to explain, "This means, for example, that if I share in a circle about my miscarriage, women don't come up to me in the tea break and share their own stories of miscarriage or offer me advice or support, unless I specifically invite them to."

This can be uncomfortable and unusual for us as listeners. We are invited not to react but just to be present and to listen with open hearts. Making an agreement not to take what is shared in the circle into follow-on conversations without the person's explicit request and permission gives us all freedom to share in the circle, even when what we choose to share is something we don't want to discuss or receive advice or help about. This principle is a boundary that creates freedom in our sharing and protects us from unwanted support and advice. It's super valuable in giving us agency over what we share, letting us each choose what we do and don't want to discuss afterwards. This is one of the boundaries that, over time, makes Red Tents feel like a brave space in which women can explore their feelings and experiences in a way that is heard and held.

In Brighton Red Tent we found it was so important to speak about confidentiality – to take the time to talk this through slowly and clearly as this piece is what will create a sense of safety for the women.

We provided the following guidelines which we spent hours and hours crafting in the Steering Circle together. As the Red Tent grew and changed, this part got longer as we realised that making this part really clear avoided awkward or tense moments later on.

We asked the women to commit to the following statement: "I commit to keep what happens here confidential. If you want to share something about what happened for yourself during a Tent you are welcome to do so, but only about yourself, not about anyone else. Other than the actual activities we do, everything else remains confidential to those present.

If someone shares something that impacts you and you have a need to speak about that elsewhere, then only share what it triggered within you and leave out all details of the person's story, so that that woman can in no way be identified.

If you want to speak to a woman during or after a circle about something she has said, ask her permission first and give her time to consider whether she wants to engage or not. Respect her decision if she doesn't wish to speak about it or receive any feedback."

Then we ask if anyone has any questions or objections to making the commitment. Thereafter we asked all present to commit to confidentiality by raising a hand.

We would then thank them and remind them that we now have a commitment, and we can remind each other of this commitment if we should forget at any time. If a woman arrives after this part briefly repeat this section to re-establish the group commitment.

Aisha

The beauty of mentioning the same things each Red Tent reminds everyone what to expect, how they can show up and ultimately that they are welcome and are invited into the space intentionally. We invite you to consider how you can make your Red Tent a brave place where you can practice what it means to speak with honesty and integrity and to hold one another in that way. You might also want to remind women that each person present is responsible for what they might want to say or not say. This means that you might choose not to share some things in the space until you are ready to share them in this kind of format. Some things you might never choose to share. At the same time, you may feel that sharing something out loud that is happening for you is helpful and legitimises your experience, as it turns it from feeling it inside to seeing it outside in the world.

[The Red Tent is] a circle of diverse and unique women where the only responsibility is for yourself and you can be wholly unreservedly authentically you. A space where women build each other up, inspire one another, support one another and grow together in an enriching circle of shared wisdom.

Emma

9.

WHAT DO YOU DO IN
THE MIDDLE?

We have a short sharing, people saying what they brought and what they need. Then whoever is holding it puts what people have shared into a big pot and cooks up how the rest of the afternoon is going to be. I think some Tents are much looser, but we are a little bit more held in that way.

Lou and Laura

Our vision and practice in Red Tent spaces has been to invite women to *be* rather than *do*. For this reason, we discourage women from over-planning too much content for their Red Tents beyond the basic structures of check-in and check-out. This is because we deliberately want to disrupt any need we might have to over-plan and instead we seek to have a simple consistent container, without a bunch of complicated activities slotted into it.

We want to make space for ourselves and for each other, and part of making that space is dispensing with an agenda of activities or things we need to get done during the Red Tent. To make this happen in the context of a Red Tent, the person holding the Tent needs to model this approach of letting go. Perhaps they might speak something that comes to their mind in the moment, perhaps they might be inspired, perhaps there is a loose theme, but what there isn't is a detailed plan and agenda. The space in between check-in and check-out is a precious space. A space to relax into.

That doesn't mean that we never do anything at all at our Red Tents! But it does mean, as someone holding a Red Tent, that we need to surrender our need to know exactly what is going to happen. This is something you have to be in the practice of. It may be challenging for you. It may also be a relief. Either way, we invite you to explore the idea that you don't need to know what will fill the time, but rather trust that it will emerge. Your role is simply to create a container in which *being* rather than *doing* is welcomed.

The structure of check-in and check-out and giving each woman a time to speak is like the banks of a river, it's what allows the rest of the time to flow. It is what creates the conditions for us to let go of *doing* and allow ourselves to *be*. It's what enables us to create a space that is more fluid than much of our lives often tend to be.

Not having a particular agenda but simply being open to what shows up on the night is very challenging, as we are all so conditioned to make things happen, rather than letting them unfold before us.
Gabriella

Sometimes we will ask the circle of women present whether there is anything they need or would like to offer into the space. They might have brought a craft activity or simply have something spontaneous, like a song, which they would like to share. And sometimes we might provide one of those offerings ourselves. But when we do, we do so without being attached to it. We offer it as a member of a collective, rather than the leader of a group.

In the event description we also said, you may wish to bring a list of suggestions, if you want to sing a song or lead an exercise or whatever. So often people did bring something that they wanted to share. But I'd say for the most part it was just talking about what's going on in our lives.
Sometimes they were more thematic: a very clear theme would emerge. Like when the Brett Kavanaugh trial was going on, a lot of women were talking about their experiences with sexual abuse and sexual trauma. [At another where a girl was] talking about birth control, pretty much the entire Red Tent ended up being about that. There was another one where somebody, one of the women who spoke first, talked about approaching 40 and still not being sure if she wanted to have kids or not. And then a lot of the women in the circle who had children or had decided not to or still wanted to [shared their experiences]. It ended up being all about motherhood and decisions about motherhood. So sometimes it stuck to

a theme, but this was very organic, and the only time that the person holding would step in was really just to keep an eye on time and wrap up, but otherwise it was pretty hands-off facilitation.

Emily

It's a bit like throwing a barbecue. You have people assembled, some things to grill, all the ingredients for a couple of tasty salads and a planned approach if someone burns a finger in the process. But the vibe, the recipes and the shape of the event is down to everyone present to co-create. And so, for us, the role of holding the Tent is not to plan out an agenda but to create the container in which there is space and flexibility. Perhaps another woman attending might suggest an activity or request some support. Perhaps others might have brought something creative they want to do together, and maybe some may simply want to rest or sleep.

Real rest within these spaces can be powerful, as can sharing our gifts in a relaxed and unplanned way. The point for us is to allow it to be unplanned, flexible and responsive to those present. We want to avoid our Red Tents becoming another area of our lives that need detailed planning and organising, we don't want to have to feel that we need to take control or direct everyone. Instead, we want to share the experience with all the women attending of a nurturing, well-held, but ultimately fluid, space.

The Beating Heart in the Centre

All this said, it does no harm to have something up your sleeve to bring to a Red Tent, even if you don't use it. As Tessa says, "Sometimes my plan goes out of the window because of something that is brought to the Red Tent on the night."

Aisha has held many Red Tents, but in the early days of holding space it felt important to have a *wireframe* of something that she could offer up to the women present. She might have the outline of an activity, the materials for it and some idea of what she might do, but at the same time she was adaptable. She didn't always actually do it!

Trust your intuition to move from one thing to another to dispel, deepen or lighten the moment with another activity. You can often feel what is needed. Trust that feeling and make suggestions to see what others feel inclined to do next. It might be the moment to stretch and move about, it might be the time to hear from someone who has brought something to read, or maybe playing some music would make sense.

Through my dark times my Red Tent Circle has been a cradle of solace into which I have fallen, always assured of a gentle landing. Through my glory days, the love of that same circle of women has never failed to lift and encourage me further. It has been a place of deep healing and growth. Through my Red Tent I have experienced the power of sisterhood and know first-hand the vital importance of it to our wellbeing.

Cali

How often do we feel honoured just for showing up?

How many times do we receive thanks for doing a million things for others?

What does it look like when we ask for help and have it met – giving us just the thing we need?

It may be that these things happen all too infrequently, or not at all. Our lives are often busy and sometimes we are not clear what we need and how to ask for it. This is where a Red Tent comes in.

We have witnessed the most extraordinary events at Red Tents of really lifting up a woman and giving her the thing she is most hungry for. We have seen women going through chemo be blessed and held in a huge hug of support. We have listened as a woman shares her sadness of losing a baby and have sat with her in that pain and each repeated a chant of: *we hear you, we see you, we love you.* We have planted seeds of hope in dark times, by holding a woman at the centre of the circle who is having a tough time and feels the bruises of life all too fresh on her skin. We have seen women use their alchemy of this collective love to express the joy they feel in other parts of their life. We have celebrated as a woman steps up, learns how to take up space when in life she feels shy, judged and marginalised. This is the power of blessing someone. This is the beauty of meeting someone in a dark corner and letting them be there, but no longer alone. This is the unspoken magic of giving someone what they need.

Angela shares with us how supported she felt by her Red Tent when she was grieving and needed a sense for consistency and a place where she didn't need to be a certain way or didn't need to present her sadness in a way that was tidy or resolved.

When my husband died Red Tent women rallied around me and held me when I asked them to. I am so grateful to the women I know, who accepted me as I am. The immediate aftermath of his death is very difficult to describe, very silent, but peaceful. As the weeks and months went by anger surfaced. I tried to keep whatever I was feeling on the surface, and not gulp it down or hide it. I didn't pretend to 'cope' or be brave. Grief, in its many forms should be outed and lived through, in my opinion. Rage, stomp, hide away, but work through it, not round it.

Angela

We wonder what a simple blessing might have looked like for her in her Red Tent. Perhaps a space to talk or to say goodbye in her own way and be witnessed in that place. This is why we need the space in the middle, as there might be a moment to fill that space with a well-needed spotlight on the parts that hurt or don't get much light. We've said about Red Tents not being a therapeutic space. They aren't. And yet collective help and support can be really healing in a collective emergent instinctive kind of way. No qualifications needed. So we suggest that you have an idea of how to offer a blessing and what that might look like so that you can offer it when needed.

What does blessing mean? What does ceremony look like? What I really like and what I sometimes say is, this is just about saying this moment really matters. And that's all it is. We're just saying this is an important moment. And that's what it means to have a ceremony. It doesn't mean we have to do anything fancy. It just means this moment matters. And I think that just keeps it really simple.

Lily

We remind you to reflect on and ask questions to understand what a particular woman would like, what they need and how the women present can offer something that resonates for them. It is really important to ask for consent in these moments in Red Tents because blessings can feel very intimate. The invitation is for a woman to be vulnerable in that situation and receive. This needs to be met with respect, time and consideration. Talking through an idea and what could be offered while checking parameters and what the person actually wants and needs is radical care for another human being. It is a rare experience to receive such a thorough implementation of consent when someone establishes your parameters with you beforehand. An additional important layer to this is ensuring there is a way to communicate, at any stage throughout the offering, if their *yes* has turned to a *no*. For example, a simple hand signal or word. This makes the act of consent a living and evolving conversation that adapts moment by moment to what is happening. It is not closing the door but clarifying permission so that if something doesn't feel right, saying so and asking for something else that does.

There's no point in rubbing her feet and singing songs if she's just going to feel really embarrassed and toe-curlingly uncomfortable and wished that she hadn't come that day. So I think that that's what I'd say: find out what she wants and make it meaningful to her.
Lily

There might also be an opportunity to share something that supports everyone as a group. A simple idea is for each woman to hold a candle and in turn lean into the centre of the circle to light the wick of their candle from the central candle while naming one woman in their life who has offered them something or reminded themselves of a quality they have but never really see.

As these simple examples show, creating a moment where you offer support at your Red Tent does not necessarily need to be a highly complex affair or a big talking session. With Red Tent spaces we can offer each other simple reminders that we are not alone and that we have a whole sisterhood of support to call in when we need to. Whether you are marking a moment in someone's life, honouring a transition or creating a way for healing to take place, you have the time to take a step towards yourselves and each other. This is the power of coming together in a Red Tent. It is how the 'empty' middle part can become the beating heart of the gathering, if there is a need and inclination that arises to meet it.

Imagine a world in which men's and women's groups held ceremonies to honour their transgender people, to welcome them into the authentic expression of their gender, like a rite of passage and a collective message of love, respect, and acceptance: "I see you, I hear you, I honour your truth". What could be more powerful? This is the future I would like to be part of. If we want to see this future become our reality, we have to take action towards it in the present moment.
Ruby

What we all want is to be accepted, recognised and loved for who we are. The thing that would mean a lot to me, I think, would be that recognition and welcome. Which is what I got mostly from women in the world around me when I transitioned and I was delighted. I think in relation to a blessing, it's more a matter of recognition. 'Hello, sister. I love to see you. I see you sister, take your place with us.'
Persia

Lots also integrate embodied practice in some way. This might include, for example, sharing meditations and visualisations, dancing or moving together and offering massage or other body work as part of a Red Tent space. Sometimes these are offered communally, in the whole circle, or other times they may happen in shared space but on an ad hoc one-to-one or one-to-many basis. Again, make sure when unplanned activities arise that there is always space for women decline taking part in an activity so that no one feels forced into doing anything that they don't want to do.

Depending on who was holding the Tent we'd start with something differ-ent. [When I lead I] do dance and embodiment a lot of the times. I start with a body flow, just breathing and checking in with all of our parts and doing a little wiggle and maybe get people moving a little bit. The others

were both musical people, they would start off with a song or a chant so we'd have some way of calling people in.
Emily

An activity can be as simple as sharing a reading or a poem. It could be a song. You might invite people to bring an activity, skill or offering that they would like to share with others in the room. We have had women bring their various creative gifts to share.

We've done craft together, with women donating odds and ends of red wool as well as spare knitting needles or crochet hooks. Each time we met women would craft while sharing and drinking tea and make small squares (15cm). We made a Red Tent red patchwork blanket that we could wrap women in if they needed extra comfort.
Su

There is a skill – and perhaps a momentum – that builds over time in creating a space in which different women are able to offer things they want to share in a Red Tent.

Woven into our sharing we have a cycle check-in, we sing, chant, medi-tate, journey, sometimes craft, sometimes we have a topic to dive deeply into, we do clothes swaps, books swaps, give massages and foot rubs, share snacks and just listen to our sisters with open hearts. I come away from each Red Tent evening feeling fed and supported on every level!
Rachael

If your Tent becomes large and many women want to make offerings this can become something that needs to be handled with care and attention. In some Red Tents this is managed by inviting women to bring things that they may wish to share, whilst being clear that there may not be the space and time for everyone's offerings at any one gathering.

Eating Together

Most Tents share food or refreshments in some way during their gatherings and sharing food can be a beautiful way of grounding the energy and connecting the group. Food, perhaps more than anything else, has so many cultural markers. It can be a wonderful way of sharing our heritage and cultures with each other, exchanging recipes as we eat together. Eating together is also a primal human act of trust and togetherness, releasing endorphins and oxytocin.

But food can also be a trigger point for many women bringing up fear, shame, guilt or discomfort. Fatphobia is an ever-present reality in our wider cultures. And our relationship to food is hugely influenced by that. This can come up when sharing food in the kinds of comments women make about themselves and what they eat or their implicit judgements about the food others eat or bring.

Meanwhile for those on restricted incomes bringing food to share might be impossible or deeply stressful. For busy working women or carers there may not be time to cook something to bring. Those who cannot cook may feel judged for their lack of home-prepared offerings.

Health conditions may also impact people's comfort in eating for example diabetes and allergies. For those with OCD, eating from shared dishes or not knowing who has touched things can be challenging and for anyone with anxiety disorders social eating can feel very out of control.

To help make the simple act of sharing food as accessible as possible in your Red Tent spaces ask those present about dietary requirements. If every woman brings something that she is able to eat, that helps ensure that everyone can be included. If food is being shared ask people to bring a label with food saying who cooked it and perhaps marking the main allergens/ restrictions: wheat, dairy, meat or specifically pork, seafood, alcohol or nuts.

You may choose to have collective guidance on food for Red Tent that is appropriate for your community and consider the needs of those attending – for example, that it must be nut free.

Be clear beforehand if there is capacity for food items that need re-frigeration, reheating or a freezer, as many venues may not have the room or facilities for this.

Be sure to have agreements on shared cleaning up and disposal of rubbish so this does not fall solely on one person's shoulders. If in a private home be respectful of the fact that the host may well not want you in her kitchen.

Be clear if there any out-of-bounds areas where refreshments cannot be taken, consumed or put down.

10.

THEMES AND ACTIVITIES

I used to use a theme quite a lot actually, because I felt like it gave direction in the circle. It helped people to have a different lens to look through what was happening in their life. And I felt like it also gave a little bit of a thread of connection between people who did or didn't know each other. Also personally it helped me to reflect differently on my experience, because I would hear someone else's completely different interpretation of that same theme.

Lily

In this section we share some ideas for themes and activities that you could use for your Red Tent. We offer them, with the proviso that if you make activities too much of the focus, Red Tents can easily start to become similar to other kinds of workshops for women. Whilst much valuable information and learning happens at those, it is not our intention to suggest that you make your Red Tent another workshop type space at all. So please always bear in mind the idea of *being*, not *doing*, and leaving space for fluidity.

Also, if you find it difficult to shake off the roar of activity then be gentle with yourself. This is also a process of unlearning the relentless 24/7 approach to productivity and 'getting things done' that you may well have learnt as early as childhood. Even if you didn't learn these particular song lyrics, then the 'look after everyone else first' anthem might be a firm favourite for you. You could also be singing both in unison or have others that are more resonant for you!

To us, the Red Tent is an opportunity to sing to your own rhythm and find the beat that pulses inside. And for people who are new to listening to the still part that exists in all of us, then you can perhaps offer a helping hand. A word of guidance or a gently offered theme or activity can sometimes lead us into a quiet place inside.

Be sure to offer clear instructions and support when setting up any theme or activity, as well as an alternative, or variation on a theme, to allow for those who might not be able, nor wish, to take part in the suggested activity.

When we do hold loose themes in our Tents, they sometimes do end up guiding the space to some extent in our check-ins, rituals, meditations, discussions and perhaps in how we decorate the centrepiece. The trick is to hold these loosely and to orient to them not as a chance to 'impart your wisdom', but as a theme around which women in the circle on a particular day can share with one another.

Sometimes we have a themed activity. That helped me in the beginning. One month we made moon bracelets. I had the wire and we made bracelets with different beads on for different stages in our cycle. We've done writing intentions. We've done burning things in the fire. We've done mood boards. That sort of thing.

I really like the idea, in time, of there being a talking seat, a bunch of women knitting and someone dozing in the corner ... In Leamington Red Tent where I went before I moved here, we'd bring lunch and share and then there might be a bit of an activity, depending on where people were at, because it was for the whole day. And sometimes I might curl up and doze while some people were crafting in the corner and someone was having a massage. It was very nourishing and nurturing.

Susannah

We have found that holding loose themes can help provide an anchor to the shape of the Red Tent, connecting us together to the time of year and some of the bigger picture things that women in the space may be thinking about. They can provide a way to explore an aspect that has come up for a number of women in a held space and above all are a fun thing to thread through the shared time and see where it goes, without needing to reach a specific destination.

In relation to these themes you will also need to be prepared to think about the needs and challenges of everyone in the room. As you read through each of the themes we explore below, you'll hopefully see what we mean by this. There is not one 'right' way to understand or engage with the topics, and so we invite you to think about holding space for exploration, rather than persuading everyone of your point of view! For us, exploring these themes is about focusing on what we share and – at the same time – understanding that not all women will have the same level of resonance with these themes.

Body

Red Tents can be a wonderful space for nurturing and appreciating bodies and so our relationships to our bodies and activities that centre on them are one of the things that you might offer in your Red Tent. But our relationships to our bodies are not always simple. We live under a capitalist system that wants to sell us solutions for all the things that we suppose might be *wrong* with us. Our bodies are a physical reminder of what it means to live in a patriarchal culture that does not value each and every body for itself. Many, many women struggle with body image and body issues. Many, many women have experienced their bodies as something to hate. Many, many women have been physically or sexually abused. Because our bodies have been such sites of abuse and critique this can be complicated to navigate.

We invite you to hold this in your awareness when thinking about body-based activities in your Red Tent, which might not feel equally comfortable for everyone. Whilst Red Tents may include aspects of embodied practice, for example, dance and meditation, we encourage you to not make assumptions about what others in the circle may – or may not – want to participate in. We invite you to consider that other people in the space might not experience them in the same way that you do.

Not everyone wants to – or can – move their body in the same way that you can.

Not everyone feels comfortable with others touching parts of their body.

Not everyone wants a massage. And not everyone wants one at the Red Tent (even if they might in private).

We invite you to consider that you may have unconsciously been holding.

For example, the idea that a thin body is a healthy body. That there is something 'good' about losing weight. That being smaller or that taking up less space is better. These are all ideas common in many of our cultures that have not always been so and that may not be 'objectively true'.

Welcoming women means welcoming their bodies and their autonomy over how they view and treat their bodies. It means welcoming their autonomy about how they want to be in their body in the space and how close or otherwise they might want other people to get to them.

We know that many Red Tents have traditions of massage which women offer one another, so we wanted to include in this part of the book a few suggestions for connective touch practices that you might offer to others in a Tent and that may feel more comfortable. While remembering always to practice consent as a principle and allowing those present to choose whether they want to participate or not in any activity that you offer. This means presenting an alternative so that there is no shame involved in opting out of an activity. It means treating someone's "no, not for me" like a precious gift that you can hold with respect, without asking for more information to substantiate their decision or trying to persuade them to try. It means being able to adapt to the needs of those present. It means letting go of an idea you have and listening to what is arising in that moment.

Hand Massage

Rather than inviting massage focused on the body, an option is to invite women to simply massage one another's hands (or even feet). This may be a very nourishing experience for some and feel more available. Please note that this doesn't mean everyone will want to take part.

Looking at One Another

Another powerful exercise that builds connection without engaging touch is to invite women, in pairs, to practice simply looking at one another. We mean really looking. Spending perhaps thirty seconds or a minute looking into one another's eyes and really seeing one another. No touch has to be involved in this, but we have found that there is a transformative power in practicing what it feels like to really see one another. Please note that this exercise may be extremely challenging, and therefore undesirable, for those on the autistic spectrum, and those with anxiety. It may also be culturally challenging for women from cultures where direct eye contact is considered rude.

Exploring Taste

Another lovely thing to do is to explore our other senses together. For example, one way to explore taste might be to share something delicious together. Have you ever tasted honey on rose petals? At the time of year when rose petals are fresh, you can pick them, add a little spoonful of honey and everyone can share in the taste almost ceremonially – together lighting up all your senses. Be sure to offer the option of not taking part in this kind of ritual to anyone who wants it.

Sex and Pleasure

We sit in circle to shine our light so that we remember what we have forgotten. We shine to celebrate the wonder of all that woman can bear, which is everything, because we are the vastness, we are the great dance of all life, fluid and changing and fully, beautifully, human.

Heidi Hinda

The Red Tent can be a place to explore sex and pleasure in our lives, yet another topic we may have rarely been invited to talk honestly about. To hold a session on sex and pleasure is to invite the women present to listen to their inner compass, the place in the body, wherever that may be, that knows what to share and how much. There are plenty of ways to bring this theme into your Red Tent so you can dip your toe in or plunge right in depending on the group.

This is a moment where practicing collective decision-making is ideal and so in creating a space for these conversations you might want to revisit confidentiality, agreements of consent and the option to not participate. As much as we can provide the space for discussions, activities or symbolic work to explore these topics, for some people they can be painful. As Zoë Le Fay reminds us, "Always hold in your mind that conversations about sex, pleasure, bodies and genitals can induce dysphoria for gender-diverse people and distress for survivors of sexual abuse."[14] Make sure you provide an alternative

---

14 With thanks to Zoë Le Fay for her support and guidance: facebook.com/StudioLeFay

activity so participating is always a choice.

Start by encouraging people to use the words and terms that resonate for them and share that there isn't a right way or wrong way to relate to or describe your body. As Barbara Carrellas articulates so well when talking about creating an inclusive space for open discussion, "Defining our terms before we speak or write is critical to accurately communicating our feelings, identities and desires."[15]

Decide what you would like to talk about together. You could talk about touch – what feels nice and why, you may want to discuss attraction and what it feels like to connect with another or you may want to share stories of significant moments for you as a sexual being. You may even want to explore how breathing can move energy around your own body and how powerful you can feel when you connect to yourself in this way.

Although our current society has a limited view of relationships as monogamous, heterosexual, single-partnered often connected through matrimony, your Red Tent doesn't need to perpetuate these as the only norm. Invite discussion about relationships which is without judgement, without assuming pronouns, without the binary frame of gender.

Exploration can happen through craft, discussion about art and images, a dialogue about language or a conversation about boundaries and where they are anchored in the body. But more than anything this is the moment to practice listening without judgement.

Sharing these conversations can help make the world a more sexually satisfied and inclusive space. Delight in what sharing conversations about sex and pleasure feel like in a held space. When discussing partners use male, female and gender non-conforming pronouns to create a culture that goes beyond the gender binary. Be mindful that the language of gender is evolving. Who we love and how we live often does not fit into neat boxes so neither need our language.

One thing we really love is the work of Colette Nolan who coined the term 'Cunt Craft', an activity which stimulates a discussion about sex, bodies, consent, boundaries, birth and everything in between. The idea is that this discussion happens while crafting: sewing or sticking materials or images together to depict your vulva, cunt, genitals (internal or external), along with a discussion of the multiple terms we use. This activity can be done as

---

15 Carrellas, Barbara. *Urban Tantra: Second Edition: Sacred Sex for the Twenty-First Century*

a solo exercise or as part of a group to encourage conversation, stories and a rich ride through language.

Colette Nolan was an ardent activist for sexual and bodily freedom and among many roles she was a sexual health educator, working with women and young people to initiate and inspire open, honest conversations about sex. She was keen on busting open gender presumptions in society and acknowledging that genitals do not equal gender. In her own words: "If you set up a space for 'women'– you set up a space for women with all types of genitals, (cocks, cunts, anything outside of that binary…) it's time to end the bitter, painful heartbreak that we inflict on ourselves every day when we contort ourselves to fit the norms."[16]

She ran numerous workshops, events, mentoring guidance, gallery events and craft sessions to empower women and gender-nonconforming people to reclaim language while reclaiming their bodies too. She was a dear friend of Aisha's and sadly died of a rare and unforgiving form of cancer in 2018. In her obituary, Lily Rose Sequoia wrote: "She faced life with a fierce and fearless passion for the deep; for the authentic; [for the humour in life]… she wasn't afraid of the dark, in fact, it's what helped her to shine."[17]

REFLECTIVE QUESTIONS

✷ What did you call the sexual parts of your body as a child, teenager, adult and how has it shaped your relationship with yourself?

✷ Drawing inspiration from Eve Ensler and her play *The Vagina Monologues,* what would this area of your body say if it could speak?

✷ If you were a caregiver for a young girl, what words would you choose now to describe parts of your body and why?

✷ How has your relationship with your own sexuality evolved through your life?

16 From Colette Nolan's blog: cherishthecunt.wordpress.com/2014/07/08/cunt-owners-are-not-always-women

17 From Colette Nolan's obituary by Lily Rose Sequoia in *She Who Knows* magazine.

Nature

Nature-based activities are very popular with Red Tents as a way to appreciate the seasons, connect to ourselves as part of the natural world or as a metaphor for talking about the cycles of our lives.

The colonisation of land and the way that nature has been abused and exploited are also themes that you might draw attention to in your Red Tent. Building a connection with the land and with nature that is symbiotic and mutually life-sustaining is not just something desperately needed in the world at this time but something you can practice in the simple activities you might engage in during your Red Tent.

If you meet near a park, wood, beach or another natural space, you might invite the women to go out and connect with the natural world to make some nature art. Invite them to see what draws their eye and to gather a small amount of fruit, nuts, bark, leaves or berries. It could be anything which is in season but, in particular, paying attention to colours, textures and shapes. When they return you could make a collective centrepiece reflecting on the season and how it is impacting them. Be sure to support those who have mobility issues.

To use nature as a metaphor you could ask women to bring something that they have gathered from nature before they come to the Red Tent: a pine cone, flower, fruit, stone, shell, nut, seeds, or vegetable. You could also gather images from magazines of nature scapes or patterns in nature. Lay them out on a cloth and ask women to choose one object or image that reflects an aspect of their life that they want to share. If women find it difficult to choose, ask them to just pick the thing that catches their eye even if they don't know why.

One woman who lives near a pebble beach brought a selection of pebbles to the Red Tent along with some acrylic paints. We painted beautiful pictures on the pebbles, words to remind us about things we had been sharing about.

Su

Tracking the Seasons

Think about this as exploring connection to the earth we live on. You might want again to draw attention to how the seasons and the cycles of nature can help us rebuild a connection with the natural world and our own place within it that has been severed by capitalism and colonisation.

Bear in mind that not all parts of the world have the same seasons, or the same definitions of season. Seasonal practices and rituals vary, and women in your circle may be bringing a very different understanding of, and relationship to, these than the one you yourself may have. We are writing from our own perspective on seasons in the UK, having also lived in other parts of Europe (Aisha) and East and Southern Africa (Mary Ann), knowing that what we share draws more on being in Northern Europe, but that some of it might be adapted to other contexts. We have tried also to provide some links to other resources that may be more relevant to your context in the references at the end of this book.

Spring: Exploring new life, new projects and new ideas. Inviting those present to share around the questions: *What is new in your life right now? What are you emerging into? Where in your life do you feel fresh and in a learning mode?*

Summer: Celebrating life in all its fullness. Inviting those present to share around the fullness of this time of year when things are in bloom: *What's blooming in your life right now? Where do you feel full? What fruits do you want to celebrate at this time?*

Autumn: Harvesting, letting go, turning inwards, focusing on the harvest of now and asking and sharing: *What are you harvesting in your life right now? Where are you grateful for fullness? What are you letting go of as this season turns to the darkness? What appreciation do we have of now that we want to bundle up and store to feast on later in the year?* When we do this, we might use a candle or piece of fruit as a talking object.

Winter: Celebrating wisdom and the darkness, writing letters and sending wishes. Invite those present to share about the darkness at this time of year and how they might resonate with it: *How do you relate to the darkness? What about winter are you grateful for? What wisdom have you gathered through the past year?*

We want to share an extended example of what this might look like in practice, taken from our own experience. We asked women to reflect on the summer solstice, considering that at this time of the year everything in nature is in its full abundance, with everything fruiting and multiplying in a rich diversity. We shared the following questions to stimulate discussion and reflection.

★ *Can you identify an aspect of this abundance that is reflected in your own life?* This could lead on to a discussion about your relationship with abundance, self-care, nurturing, and nourishment.

★ *Can you share something you have observed as you stopped to pause recently?* This could lead on to exploring your senses with a shared moment of quiet or passing around objects in small bags that represent smell, sound or touch.

★ *What of this time full of light with long days would you like to take with you into the darker months, to remember at that time?* This could lead to writing a letter to yourself at the winter solstice and one person in the group could offer to post these out to women in mid-winter.

Cycles

This section includes a range of activities that connect us to the cyclical natures of our lives, bodies and planet.

Life Cycles

I love it when we get women of all different ages, young and old, from various walks of life. It's a gift to hear and learn from all women. It helps me to reflect, to grow and to love more! I leave the Red Tent with heightened senses, seeds of ideas, small wishes for myself, feeling hugged and cosy.

Mads

Many times in Red Tent spaces things we could describe as relating to our life cycles come up. These might include conversations about things we – or women in our circle – may not often talk publicly about, including conversations about menstruation and our first bleeding experiences; about female genital mutilation, sexual violence and abuse; conversations about sex, sexuality, identity, forced marriage, pregnancy, baby loss, infertility and menopause; conversations about ageing and illness and death.

The many lived experiences of women are as diverse as there are women to have them. This list isn't exhaustive and no one running a Red Tent can – or should feel like they need to – be an expert in all of these. It is more a case of having an awareness of holding an inclusive, non-judgemental space for sharing and listening to each other.

A Red Tent is where there are shared strands of experiencing motherhood. I think that's where value is because everyone's life and choices are different. I want to learn from women who've birthed their babies, as much as I hope they want to learn from me as a woman who hasn't.
Lu

As women begin to realise that they can share honestly, without fear, that they will not receive responses unless requested, you will likely find more and more reflections and experiences about these things will begin to be shared.

In our circle we have heard stories of loss, break ups, cancer, divorce, miscarriage, pain and heartache, we have celebrated conceptions, births, marriages, menopause, end of breastfeeding…and all the passages of womanhood you can imagine! I come away from each Red Tent evening feeling fed and supported on every level!
Rachael

It can be useful, therefore, to have resources and ideas about some of these themes to hand in case they become useful in your Red Tent space. This might happen in a relatively impromptu way, or you may find that it works best if you plan this a little so that you are prepared.

At one of my favourite Red Tents, a sixteen-year-old came, having seen the Tent shared on Facebook. She showed up on her own and she said, "My doctor said I should go on the pill. And I'm just wondering, you know, about birth control? I want to hear from different women about what they do or did." And it was amazing, because we had a circle of women from age sixteen to seventy that day, and everyone was really clear about talking from their own experience.

Emily

Through Red Tents we have learnt time and time again that not everyone experiences life cycles in the same way. So think about using open questions that allow women to share what their own real experience is. Open questions are questions that could have a multitude of different answers depending on someone's circumstance and don't lead the answer into a narrow box. For example:

★ Where are you in the cycles of your life?

★ What grief have you known as a woman?

★ What about the age you are now strikes you?

★ What are you seeing in yourself at this stage in your life cycle?

★ How do you feel about this stage in your life cycle?

★ How do you relate to others from this place in your life?

★ What is changing in your life, in your body, at this point in your life cycle?

Birth and Death

You might also want to create themes around birth and death or enable women to share stories about being born, giving birth, death or about loss and grief. We recommend some resources in our resource section to help with this[18] and also invite you to choose carefully being aware that not all women want to or are able to birth children and that not everyone may wish to share about issues like grief and death. However, everyone has both been born and will die, so you can open it from this perspective and welcome everything in between. This can be such fertile ground for sharing within the model of witnessing people without response. It can bring up a lot and honest sharing about these things can have a healing quality if your questions invite a whole diversity of answers. This is where creating brave spaces where difference can live is really crucial. And it's also not without challenge, as we will explore more deeply in the next section.

You might invite women to reflect together on questions such as:

✷ What do you know of your own birth experience? (Remember that some women may have no knowledge about this, in particular those who might have been adopted or separated from the person who birthed them.)

✷ Who or what have you birthed in your life? How did you celebrate it?

✷ Who and what have you lost in your life? How did you grieve it?

Note to self

One way to reflect is to use writing as an activity. It can be a way to honour the knowledge and wisdom that we have for ourselves. You can each write a letter to your sixteen-year-old self from the perspective of being an adult now and what you have learnt, or advice you imagine from an older, wiser self to you now. What do you need to hear? What do you need to say?

Be mindful of those who may struggle with writing and suggest that speaking into their phone to capture it as a voice message might be a possible alternative. Other people prefer to draw to express their response to a prompt. Make clear that people can write or express themselves in the language or creative format they feel most comfortable using, and that there will be no

---

18 See in particular *Outside the Box – Everyday Stories of Death, Bereavement and Life* by Lizzie Rothshild and *Saying Goodbye* by Zoe Clark-Coates.

pressure to share these with the group.

The person holding the Red Tent might offer to post these out to those in the group at a date in the future, ensuring that they are sealed and not opened by anyone before this date. Alternatively, people can take them home to read again later or destroy them as part of the process. If you are meeting online, someone could take responsibility for receiving them by email and sending them back to people on a future date. Be sure to share an agreement as to what will happen with them before you begin the exercise.

Lunar Cycles

Perhaps since the very beginning of humanity, in many cultures and contexts, we have felt a resonance with and seen our own reflection in the moon. And so, sharing about our awareness of moon cycles can offer one way to explore the meaning of cyclical nature in our lives. For example:

✸ What resonance (if any) do you feel with the moon?

✸ What do you notice about how you feel when the moon is dark?

✸ What do you notice about how you feel when the moon is full?

Menstrual Cycles

When you invite women to share about cycles some will want to share about their menstrual cycle and their relationship to it. In *The Red Tent,* the original book by Anita Diamant, the women of the novel went into a Tent to bleed together. For many women the Red Tent is a recreation of this time and a reminder that rest and relaxation nourish us if and when we bleed.

But always remember that not all of us in any circle will bleed and also that we are not all bleeding on the same schedule and there is no one schedule of the moon on which it is better or worse to be bleeding. Some women – at any one meeting – may be bleeding, others may be ovulating. Many who attend Red Tents don't bleed, no longer bleed or don't currently have periods for a whole host of different reasons.

If a Red Tent event is centred on menstruation, or ones that refer directly to biological processes – attendees can make an informed decision on whether or not to attend, and leave if they need to; this applies to both cisgender and transgender women.

Olivia

That doesn't mean we can't talk about periods, but what we need to be aware of is that not everyone shares the same lived experiences. Not talking about menstruation has been a way of us honouring the shame attached to it under patriarchy. But assuming everyone has the same lens as you can also narrow our vision and exclude people from the many diverse experiences and perspectives that make up our lives as women.

At the Red Tent that was set up in my local area recently, there was a goddess every month. A goddess that was chosen and stipulated by the organiser, which is something that I find really challenging. It's really presumptuous suggesting that I would have anything to bring to that and it made me feel uncomfortable. It's important to pay attention to the cultural aspects of choices, to avoid all of that blurring that can happen under 'spirituality'...

Lu

We are not sharing in the Red Tent so that we all feel or think the same. Quite the opposite, we are sharing our differences, our own challenges, our own learnings. Not to force them on other people but to have a place to be witnessed and heard in our own journey. In another's story we might find threads of our own or we might find ourselves thinking, our experience is nothing like that. All of that is welcome. We don't come to be made the same but to honour and witness our differences and to share our experiences with one another.

Who am I? Where am I from?

Naming who we are and our stories about where we are from and our own ancestry can be an important component of bringing into awareness our cultural heritage. A simple prompt could be to invite each woman to share something about where she is from and perhaps some stories from home, whatever that means for her.

Matrilineal Lines

On these islands, the United Kingdom, we live in a culture that has traced inheritance down the paternal line, with women often changing from their father's to their husband's surname when they marry. In this way the matrilineal name and identity is erased in our naming traditions, though of course some people choose to resist this. Naming traditions vary around the world. In some places women do keep their name, but many are patriarchal in this way.

The first time I was married I participated in a naming ceremony and was given a new name by the family that I had married into. Thereafter they never uttered my birth name again but knew me by the name they had given me. I was from a different background and so the custom was new for me. I did feel a sense of welcome but also had this uneasy feeling like I had somehow been erased at the same time.

Margot

The following exercise deliberately brings awareness to our matrilineal line and the names of the women that came before us. It allows us to ask ourselves what threads of those past women and their life stories we carry in our lives. It asks us to think about what we have inherited, what we want to change in our lifetime and what we want to pass on to the next generation either as parents, mentors or carers.

✴ I am Aisha, daughter of Rosie, granddaughter of Stella.

✴ I am Mary Ann, daughter of Jean, granddaughter of Eveline Joan.

✴ I look at the women in my family and the qualities I see that I want to embrace are...

✴ I look at the women in my family and the challenges they faced that I want to address in my lifetime are...

Who Were my Ancestors?

This is one way in which you can seek to bring attention to histories of racism, slavery and colonisation into your Red Tent space by asking people to share what they know of their ancestors. You can specifically invite people to share how white supremacy and racism show up in what they know about their family or origin or ancestry. They can also share how liberation shows up.

For many people, this will bring a combination of different realisations. Some harm and complicity, some pain and grief, some resistance they can lean in to. You can hold this in the same way that you hold the rest of the Red Tent as a circle with women sharing for a few minutes each.

You can do this with a mixed group but be aware that white women sharing about the complicity of their ancestors in racism, slavery and white supremacy may be unnecessarily painful and burdensome to those who have experienced racism their whole lives, even if some of these stories also exist in their own heritage. This might be an opportunity to create separate spaces for a period of time – perhaps in different rooms where white women share with one another and Black women and other women of colour share their own stories. You might then come together and share what you have learnt.

Creating dedicated spaces for the purposes of exploring the impact of racism and our complicity in it has a long tradition in racial justice work in the United States. The aim is not to create separate paths, so much as to find ways to explore the topic which unites those with shared experience. They can create a healing space for women who have experienced racism and a space for white people to investigate their own identity and ancestry as a source of motivation in taking action for racial justice without further traumatising people of colour.

Girl Time

A Red Tent can be a place where we discuss aspects of our lived experiences when we were growing up, the socialisation of being a girl and the ways that shaped us at the time and now on reflection. It can also be a place we create for the next generation. As Carly, a former member of our Red Tent

Directory team, used to say, "it takes a village," when she was reflecting on raising her two daughters. The idea of nurturing a community to be that metaphorical village has inspired many women who organise Red Tents.

It came about because I wanted to attend a Red Tent but there wasn't one near to me that I could feasibly get to with young children (the youngest was 18 months old). So I thought that I knew a few women who'd be interested and would give it a go! The vision was that my daughters would have an established Red Tent community to support them as they grew up. Over the years of running the Red Tent, I've heard so many women wish that they'd had this knowledge and support much earlier and so I wanted to take this directly to the girls so they didn't have to wait!

Tessa

To me, Red Tent means to re-create a support village for the future generations of women. Restore rites of passage ceremonies to support us through the change. As a doula, I recognize the importance of the transition from being a woman to being a mother, and as a mother, I want for my daughter to rediscover the support group during her growth phases, and to learn how to better know herself.

Tamara

I don't know if I'm doing this for my daughters. There's a bit of me that wonders whether I would want for there to always be a need for a Red Tent, because is there only a need for them because patriarchy has gripped and defined our lives for so long? But then again I sort of immediately second guess that because it's not just about a safe place, it's that there's a different quality to interaction somehow, sitting with people who have a shared experience, an experience of being a woman, whatever that means, and that is delicious and nourishing in some way that is really hard to describe.

Lu

REFLECTIVE QUESTIONS

★ What were you hungry for when you were growing up and how could that have been met?

★ What are your hopes and vision for girls living in the world today?

★ What makes a resilient community that we can all be a part of creating?

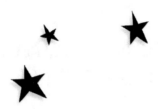

PART FOUR

11.

CHALLENGES, CONFLICT AND GROWTH

Instead of looking at each other with eyes of correction – 'I've got to fix you, I've got to make you better in some way, I've got to teach you what you don't know which I also didn't know last week' – there's just this way that we look at each other in movement that is not loving and I wanna figure out how we return to that like, 'you get to be here and be whole here and be loved here' and that requires a lot of accountability.

adrienne maree brown [1]

The Red Tent movement is a term that describes many different women meeting in many different ways in many different countries. We hope it is clear by now that Red Tents are not in any way a co-ordinated group of gatherings, but rather women doing something for themselves together in their communities. At the Red Tent Directory, although we list Red Tents around the world, we don't control, approve, or organise them.

Not all spaces called Red Tents will look or feel like what we have been describing in this book and you could call yours something different while it may reflect some of the elements we have discussed. But we are writing to invite you to think about running your gathering collectively in a way that promotes liberation and we know that doing that will mean challenges, it will mean tricky moments, it will mean getting things wrong. It will also

---

1   adrienne maree brown on *Finding Our Way* podcast with Prentis Hemphill, "Episode 2 – Visioning with adrienne maree brown"

mean changing your mind and things not going to any kind of perfectly formed plan. Accountability and a willingness to change is, as adrienne maree brown suggests, what makes being whole and loveable in shared space possible.

In this section we want to share some examples of the challenges and conflicts that can come up in Red Tent spaces and some tools for navigating these tough situations, dynamics and conversations.

In our view, the fact that problems appear to be surfaced, named and addressed is one of the markers of holding community with integrity. That's why we encourage you to nurture courageous collective leadership that isn't afraid to deal with the challenges and conflicts that may arise in your Red Tent. Over our time supporting Tents to address these kinds of issues, we have developed some approaches that, though they won't necessarily prevent challenges from arising, we hope will help you to navigate them when they do.

We firmly believe that, rather than hoping that you have found a magic formula for community that will unfold easily and harmoniously forever, it is better to build collective structures that equip you to address challenges as and when they arise. Because they will. And learning to be a Red Tent space that can work with and explore conflict and disagreement is what we believe will strengthen your Red Tent as a community-space for the longer term.

It takes work and intention to ensure that collectively held space is open, accountable, inclusive and resilient. It goes along with what we have already shared about Red Tents being intentional, about developing anti-oppressive and liberatory practices and seeking to grow safer spaces alongside the acceptance that at times conflict and disagreement will arise.

In the Red Tent Directory we receive a number of requests for support from women who are dealing with issues that arise in Red Tents. We welcome these requests. Asking for help is so important. If a doubt or issue arises that you feel you don't have the skill set to resolve or the experience to draw on, then we also encourage you to appeal to your wider circle of connections for support. Often it is how you respond to this that makes the difference and the most important thing to remember when dealing with challenges is that you are unlikely to be the first group to ever experience one of this type.

Examples of Challenges
and Conflict in Red Tent Spaces

There are many issues which can arise and unsettle the peaceful flow of your gatherings. We want to share just a few examples we have seen and heard about. We share them to help you prepare for and navigate challenges and conflict that may come up for you. We are all learning and unlearning together. A later section will deal with some ways of resolving these issues.

Challenges around Finances

Earlier in this book we have shared our vision for Red Tents as free or donation-based, community spaces. But we are steeped in a capitalist culture and so this doesn't always happen easily. Some women do choose to charge for Red Tent spaces as a way to be compensated for their energy. This in turn can feel challenging to those who feel the dynamics of the space are altered with this monetary exchange. We have learnt that the free and donation-based model only feels good if there is genuinely a collective approach rather than a situation in which one woman feels she carries the burden so that everyone else can experience the space.

Example 1

How can we sit in circle, completely free and equal, if some women are ticket-holding customers and others have been paid? How can we ensure that a Red Tent is as open and accessible to all women, if they have to find £10 for the cheapest ticket? And how can there be justification for the use of these funds, even before the group itself has begun? I wanted so much to support this – how could I not, it having been such a long-held dream? – and so I duly paid my fee and joined the first meeting as a reluctant 'customer'. I came away feeling frustrated and sad. Nurtured by some wise and dear friends, I've resolved to set up another circle to meet my needs and those of amazing women in my community. I hope that the vision can form itself in a gentler and more organic way.

Example 2

Red Tent meetings don't happen in a vacuum, they happen in a culture where women are expected to self-sacrifice: to not value or invest in ourselves, to bear the burden so others are free from that, to rescue others at our own expense. And so the mistake that I made with the Red Tent was to hold the ethos that it should be free or donation-based, but also juggle that with the fact that we wanted to remove power dynamics and create a neutral space, which meant paying for a venue. This meant that costs needed to be met, so while some women could afford to donate, others could not, which led to me holding the majority of the financial burden. We moved venues to a place where we could 'donate' to the venue costs, but then I felt a responsibility to ensure that this 'gift' was not taken advantage of, so I would top up the donations to reflect what I thought the space was worth. So the Red Tent was free for everyone... except me! I have mixed feeling about it now. I feel like yes, Red Tents should be free, and I also feel like we still have a way to go in terms of our relationship with economics, exchange, self-value and self-sacrifice before this can be done in a healthy way.

Conflict with Other Local Red Tents

Sometimes a Red Tent starts up on what feels like another Red Tent's 'patch' and there is conflict about whose space it is, who was first or has the right to use a name of a particular geographical area.

Example

Another group insisted on their uniqueness and that they run the real, traditional Red Tent. But it's not about tradition. It is about responding to the needs of the community. I offered to run the Red Tent together with the woman who started the other group, but she didn't want to. I figure we both have something to offer and that the group I have created will speak to women in different ways.

Conflict Between and Amongst the Group

Red Tent spaces are also spaces in which – as we've explored earlier in the book – we can be triggered and conflict can emerge amongst the group.

Example

We realised we needed to know each other much more in order to trust each other. We needed to have some joint experiences and we started to work on that. But quite early on, there were people getting triggered in the circle and so it was this amazing experiential learning of, "Okay, so now we need to introduce a way of talking clearly about the situation we see, how we are feeling and what we want to resolve together." Various challenges happened within our circle. It would be fine for a bit and everyone was sort of like, "Oh, this is great," and then suddenly – maybe it's just a one-to-one trigger, or it's triangled within that circle and you're observing that triangle, then you're being pulled towards the different elements and needing to hold that.

Sharing Leadership – Really Sharing it!

Sometimes as Tents grow and change, a conflict can also signal the need for a change in how you organise your Red Tent or the holding structure that you use.

Example 1

Attendance was dwindling and willing volunteers to host were not coming forward. I stepped up as part of the group to form the holding circle because I knew from first-hand experience the power of this sacred space for women. If we had not created the holding circle group, I believe the strong legacy of our Red Tent would have come to an end.

If the responsibility lies on a few shoulders for an extended period of time it can take the shine off being involved. Ideally you want to be able to host a Tent and then the next month lean back and experience the full holding of one so that you too get to fill up.

Example 1 [part 2]

Our holding circle is our saving grace and having four of us in the group means that each of us can step in to hold the actual Red Tent from time to time without feeling overwhelmed, and, that we get the delight of meeting one another periodically. It has been a complete joy for me. And especially because it means that if one of us needs to take a rest, there are three others holding.

When this doesn't happen it can impact on the wellbeing of the one or few people doing a lot of the organisation and arranging.

Example 2

People didn't want to join the steering circle, I think perhaps it was the work aspect that people didn't like. They loved the Red Tent and wanted to extend that feeling into their life and to be a greater part of it and then as soon as they found out that there were kind of hard tasks involved they left as soon as they could and that was very difficult.

My part in that was that I wanted to support my love and passion and how it really transformed me as a woman. And I just couldn't let the ball go because it was too important to me. So I suppose the first task that was dropped I picked it up, the second task that was dropped, I picked up and all of a sudden it felt like I was juggling everything. I put myself in that position. I kept on making that choice until I got to the point of just saying to myself, "You know what, I really have to trust now that if I don't do this, somebody is going to do it."

Example 3

My hope was that over time the women would value the space and want to invest time and energy into making it happen. They would feel called to offer their own flavour to the Tent. They would feel inspired to offer a theme, or suggestion. To offer to host or facilitate. I had a vision that over time it would grow into a healthy and sustainable community. In reality, this did not happen as I had hoped. In truth, I began to resent being the one to hold the Red Tent alone. I loved seeing women value the space I had created, but I wished that I had that too.

Every Tent I would ask women to volunteer to help sustain it. I tried various different strategies: suggesting that they 'hold a section' – perhaps sharing a craft, supporting a discussion or holding a ritual. I offered to mentor – to help women plan for the next Tent. We explored what barriers were stopping women stepping forward and how we could remove those barriers (was it the location, venue, timing, finances, confidence?). We worked through lots of: 'not good enough', 'I'm too busy', 'this is my only respite, I don't want responsibility'. We developed many solutions. Some women did step forward to offer little bits, but it felt like they were doing it as a favour to me, rather than as a way of contributing and investing in a space they valued to make the Tent sustainable. It's clear to me now that to be sustainable the Red Tent needs to be a collaboration.

Example 4

I am a holder of Red Tents, but there's a strong part in me that doesn't want people depending on me to be the leader. So I have a kind of paradox or relationship with this leadership because, for me, every woman can lead a Red Tent and yet they will not run a Red Tent without seeking my consent. I have a certain resistance to setting up anything that is always the same. I want each one to be different. But they love it. They love being led. But I have a resistance to always leading. You can do a Red Tent this way and this is the way I do it. But I think we all have our own innate creativity and I feel quite strongly about that.

Example 5

My vision for it was that it was a shared thing. That we shared leadership, shared hosting. But that's not what happened. Maybe one or two people stepped up that year. Every month I'd ask, "Does anybody else want to hold the group and we'll help you, I'll sit with you and I'll give you the kind of framework or structure, and then you can do whatever you want. You don't have to do it the same way. These are just basic precepts…". It actually took until I was seven months pregnant and saying, "I'm not going to be able to lead this anymore." And then someone stepped up. Other people started to do it. And it was great. Now people are stepping up and holding them I think the pressure is off me as well because what was happening was because I kept doing it every month, I was almost starting to ingrain a style into it, which was my style, and I didn't want it to be that, I wanted it to feel collaborative.

Example 6

For me, it's been a revelation in how to move away from the patriarchal pyramid with one or two people making a decision from above. At the start, we were sort of at the top, because we founded it and someone has to start. And then it got to a point where there was some jostling within the holding circle and people wanted to be more involved. And one day – which we laugh about now – one of the women said, "Well, you've asked us to join in. Don't you want us to help you?" And that was the paradigm shift for me because it was a letting go of something that the two of us had set up and steered a particular way. And stepping back and thinking to myself, "We are all now going to be doing this equally. And that's going to mean that I'm going to be overruled sometimes." It was a leap of faith, a sort of jumping into the dark with it all and trusting that we could do this collectively. Letting go. And a little bit of ego having to be thrown out because it was now going to be community-owned. It's been a very good learning curve.

Example 7

You can't just negate what people are feeling and what's going on in their lives and just run the Red Tent, because otherwise you're not including everything that's going on within the circle. It just doesn't work. It's extremely deep work. People have been triggered and dealt with very deep core issues in the circle. It's been amazing the evolution that we've all gone through, and some people in particular. What some people have been supported through has been really remarkable.

But there's definitely been times when there's a lot of emotional stuff coming up in a circle, there's all these challenges and sometimes you just think, "Ahhh!

I've got my own life to lead." But we also know that it's our own feelings. And so, just being able to hold that, and keep going, and just know that it will get easier. I've been through a lot of my own stuff and evolved hugely through being in the circle, learning a lot about how you hold a circle and hold your own stuff as well. Two things parallel and having to practice that.

Challenges About How the Red Tent is Run

Sometimes challenges may emerge from different dynamics that show up in your Red Tent space. Not everyone takes the same approach to Red Tents. There are some things we have advocated for in this book for example, that some Red Tents may be doing differently. For us, making time for sharing and allowing what naturally emerges in the group is what makes Red Tents a different way of connecting than a training session or time specific activity, as does holding the space in a way that is different to an unstructured informal chat. But other approaches also may be offered and you may find conflict emerges about the best way to hold and run your gatherings.

Example 1

When I first started, I was co-hosting with a woman who does feminine wisdom-type work, but it was way too facilitated. We were sitting in a circle, but it was all about her sharing her wisdom and guiding women through all these different things. I feel that in general we are over-programmed. For me that's a part of this masculine imbalance in our society: everything is structured and programmed and you go into an event and there's a clear objective and we're going to hit these criteria and you know, by the end of this workshop you will know x, y, z. And I wanted this to be a space for embracing the mystery, in a spirit of co-creation, where you don't really have expectations other than, you know, I'm just going to show up and be real and see what happens. So I had to tell that woman: "Look, I really just want this to be about the people in the circle."

Example 2

Lots of effort had clearly gone into the planning of the afternoon. So much so that it felt non-stop, with three led 'activities', a brisk pace, and no opportunity for checking in or open sharing from the whole group. Almost 20 women showed up, wonderfully, but despite the carefully printed name stickers and feedback sheets, I never got to hear from each of them. In experiencing this group session, I came away feeling frustrated and sad.

Example 3

Challenges that arose were very occasional. In my experience, we once had a very distressed woman looking for support, help and answers and a lot of the evening was taken up by her situation. Of course, we are all there to help and love, but as holder of the space it is our role to keep the container held and for there to be space for all women. On that occasion, many others did not have the time to share what they needed to.

As this woman shared it can be challenging to hold a space in which someone is particularly distressed and needs more support than is available in a Red Tent space. On these occasions you, of course, have to hold the space as best you can. This is the time to suggest additional support, perhaps sharing details of other services which the person could access locally to assist them during a difficult time. As the following woman shares, there may also be a need to remind new people of guidelines.

Example 4

A very strong personality came and took a lot of space, and that was a bit of a challenge because I tend to hold space quite gently and set quite clear rules and boundaries at the beginning and say, you know, this is what this space is for. I guess I'm lucky that I normally work with people who respect the space of other people. Different personalities always pop up. But she took up quite a lot of space, and I didn't want to squash her. But I wonder if I should've just kerbed her slightly. So that's a bit of learning.

Example 5

The way that the group was structured was that it was closed for two sessions and open for one session, so that in the closed group there was space for deeper exploration with the same people present. That is how I had structured it.

Then one day I had a long chat with a woman who was going through some stuff and I said, "Look, why don't you come to the Red Tent? I think it'd be really good for you." We have this WhatsApp group, and I said, "It's not an open group this month but I'll just ask everyone if you can come, I'm sure it'll be fine."

So I went into the WhatsApp group added her to the group and introduced her to everyone. But someone said, "It's a closed group this month," and a big discussion followed while this new woman was on the thread and then she ended up leaving the thread and saying, "Look I just don't really need this right now and I'm just not going to come. Don't worry about it." I was left feeling really awkward, and it also meant that I had compromised my relationship with the other people in the group because I had unwittingly said, "Oh, yeah, of course it's okay to change the rules because it's my group, I've been setting the rules so far, so I can be flexible on them."

I had the intention of checking in with everyone, but I shouldn't have added her to the WhatsApp group beforehand. So the learning there was about not adding someone to the group without them actually having been to a session. The second thing we agreed was no discussions on WhatsApp, only using it for facts and information about sessions. And the third thing was if you're going to change a rule, you need to do it in person with the group first, not over WhatsApp. And finally, if you've got rules, you just need to follow them.

Because what ended up happening is that she ended up feeling unsafe, and so did everyone else in the group. And even though about 80% were happy with her joining, there were a couple of people in particular who really didn't want that to happen. So it was a really big lesson.

What I did was I contacted everyone personally who was engaged with it, and just said, "Look, I totally get where you're coming from. Let's try and sort out." So we held a circle to do so.

It's worth talking about conflict, because it's actually part of the Red Tent. It's an important point, I think.

What came out of it is that we would hold a vote for the group to decide whether it was going to be open or closed [to new members]. But we decided that night that we wouldn't change anything until the end of the year. So that's what we did. And now it's always open.

And actually, it's always the same people that come anyway. It didn't really make a massive difference. It was more about having agreed guidelines. And I would recommend that each group create their own document of what the rules are going to be and that it gets reviewed regularly, because groups flex and change.

I also learned that when you set the rules for the group, everyone has to stick to the rules, and if you want to change the rules, everyone has to agree to do so: there has to be a democratic or consensual process that enables the change.

Conflict Around Welcoming Trans Women and Non-Binary People to a Red Tent

As the next woman shares with us, welcoming trans women and non-binary people to a Red Tent can bring up issues if the appropriate preparation and discussion has not been put in place as we recommend. As you'll read in this piece, she discussed whether to welcome trans women and non-binary people to a Red Tent space she had created, and there was disagreement amongst the group.

We must emphasise that trans women have a right to participate in women-only spaces because they are legally women and are therefore afforded the rights based on their gender. As we shared earlier in the book, we suggest that you take leadership on this and be clear why it is important to welcome all those identifying as women, both cis and trans and non-binary individuals to Red Tent spaces.

When I started the group we had four women that came regularly, including myself, for a few months… We had a Facebook page and it was open to anyone who wanted to come along. We had a lot of women joining the Facebook group but then not coming to any Red Tents. I think we didn't really think about it until I got a message from a woman, who had joined the Facebook group and never been to a Red Tent saying, "What's your policy on including trans women? I really don't think they should be allowed into women-only spaces and I think you need to have a policy on it."

I brought it up in a Red Tent. And my honest reaction to that was, "This is ridiculous, this woman hasn't even been to one of our groups and she's trying to tell me that we should have policies and what those policies should be." It felt like an imposition and we all sort of felt that we would just cross that bridge when we came to it and that we didn't need to think about it particularly in advance.

Then a person who had just joined our Facebook group who identified as non-binary and was assigned male at birth said that they would be coming to one of our events. So then this opened up a conversation about what we were going to do. What we came to was that it didn't make sense for us to have a non-binary person in a women's circle because by defining it as a women's circle, we're saying that we feel that there are these two genders. A non-binary person by definition is someone that rejects those genders and so we just didn't see the fit.

And then we talked about whether we'd let in trans women. And I started by saying that if someone identifies as a woman, then I'm okay with them coming. But another woman in my group argued quite strongly against it. She made the argument, which made sense to me at the time, that a trans woman was someone who had been born and grown up with male privilege in a patriarchal society benefitting from a sense of entitlement that comes so naturally to people that are born male.

I was like, "Okay, yeah, that makes sense. I understand that somebody that's born male will grow up with a completely different perspective to us, even if that person then later identifies as female." So we decided that our policy was going to be that we were only open to women that were born as women.

We didn't tell the non-binary person that we'd made a decision. We just sort of left it and they never got in touch again.

But after that Red Tent meeting, I started going to a lot more queer events. (I identify as bi-sexual and always have done, but I had been in a straight relationship for four or five years which had just ended.) I met some trans women and non-binary people at these events. As soon as I started talking to trans women I soon realised that they had not grown up in a position of male privilege at all. They were very much othered. When I was speaking to trans women, I had an instant feeling of recognition and connection that here is someone else that understands what it's like to grow up in a patriarchal society as another oppressed person. That we have that in common.

One time I was speaking to a trans woman and realised I would be horrified if they knew I was part of a women's group that was not allowing trans women in. That I don't want to be a part of something that I feel ashamed of. I'm not okay with this. From that point on, the Red Tent became less of a support for me and more of a problem. It was a bit of a liability, in a way, because I didn't want to be identified with a group that was excluding people. For me, what defines my experience of being a woman, is my experience of being oppressed and being othered. The fact that I share that experience with trans women makes me happy to have that person in circle with me.

I would like to live in a world where gender doesn't matter, where everybody could be non-binary and free to express more so-called masculine or feminine qualities, or whatever mix is right for them. I think that would be amazing. For me, it's always been a struggle against feeling pushed into a box and being pressed into a particular role and trying to fight against that. To try to be seen as a person rather than a gender.

REFLECTIVE QUESTIONS

✴ What resonated with you or challenged you about the stories and examples shared? Why do you think this is?

✴ What sensations did you experience in your body as you read this section?

✴ What would you do if you experienced situations like these, perhaps drawing on your own resources and the guidance you have read in this book?

✴ What agreements and discussions would you like to put in place to create safer spaces and ones where conflict is an opportunity for growth?

Resolving Conflict and Building Liberatory Accountability

Because of the way we have been trained and shaped by punitive sys-
tems…we really wanna be innocent and so we will reject the information
we are getting about our own behaviour because it disrupts who we want
to be or think we are and we'll do everything we can to paint the scene so
that it removes any of our culpability or responsibility or accountability
in it. So I think the other side of the culture shift that's necessary is for
it actually be – for lack of a better word – safe enough to care about the
impact that you have had on another person but also to have it instilled
in us that it matters. That we are impacting each other all the time and
that it does matter when we – in our own unconsciousness or our own
unprocessed things – transgress or cross boundaries or cause harm. That
has to really matter.

Prentis Hemphill [2]

Most challenges require courage to resolve. You will likely need to stretch
beyond your comfort zone and get busy with some discomfort in order to
move forward. Few of us have been taught how to resolve conflict produc-
tively, and we can really struggle with being in or around conflict. But learning to be with conflict while processing and moving through it is one of the
things we need to learn as we build community together: it is the only way
through to a more liberatory way of being together.

Consider for a moment the conversation that has been initiated in the US
by Black Lives Matter around defunding the police. Their analysis is that the
system that is meant to resolve problems and keep society safe is not working. It is causing Black people more harm. It is making them less safe. And
they make the point therefore, there is a need for a new system, a new way
of addressing and preventing and making amends for harm.

If we want to create spaces where we can be together in new ways we too
will ultimately have to face the question of:

---

2 *Finding Our Way* podcast with Prentis Hemphill, "Episode 2 – Visioning with
adrienne maree brown"

What do we do when things become difficult between us?

What do we do when there is harm?

How can we stay accountable? And what does repair look like?

How can we address problems head-on without falling apart? Without losing each other? Without condemning each other?

How do we do that in a way that is just? And that invites liberation rather than in a way that closes down difference or re-perpetuates harm?

Building our tools for dealing with conflict and becoming accountable, for allowing change to happen between us and in how we relate to one another is part of this work of liberation. It's the messy and difficult practice that helps bring into reality the bolder vision we have for this work.

Meanwhile, for many of us addressing conflict may be traumatic, meaning that it may remind us of difficult experiences that we may have had in the past and it may therefore trigger reactions in us that are subconscious. This means that, whilst we may want to resolve problems, we may find ourselves instead quickly adopting a response that comes from the part of our brain designed to keep us safe from danger. This may lead us to fight back, freeze and not know what to do next, fly away and disconnect completely, or to please others in an attempt to just stop the conflict from happening and get out of the way. All of these responses are patterns that we can find ourselves stuck in and in our experience, often do. They are a response to a threat system in the part of our brains that we share with other animals. They are reasonable responses to actual physical threat, of course. But they don't help us to navigate conflict when our bodies sense threat that may no longer be actively present. Rather they often exacerbate it. To move to a different response we often need to calm our nervous systems first:

Ease back into your body. Fear launches us into "heady" worrying, or numbing and spacing out. Gently ask your body to relax. Feel each of your major muscle groups and softly encourage them to relax. (Tightened musculature sends unnecessary danger signals to the brain.) Breathe deeply and slowly. (Holding the breath also signals danger.) Slow down. Rushing presses the psyche's panic button... Feel the fear in your body without reacting to it. Fear is just an energy in your body that cannot hurt you if you do not run from it or react self-destructively to it.

Pete Walker [3]

Having followed these steps it is often also helpful to move your body in some way that helps it to discharge any energy that remains. [4]

As Sarah Peyton says about resolving conflict with each other and within ourselves, "As we become better able to regulate ourselves, we become more resilient, less reactive, and more stable. At the level of our body, we begin to stay more grounded, easily experiencing what used to upset us without losing our neuroception of safety... As we feel safe, we use words in ways that let others feel safe, too. Our bodies relax together as the patterns of communication shift and we learn to take more responsibility for our thoughts, our words, our actions." [5]

With these tools in mind, we want to reflect on what happens in practice in your Red Tent. One Red Tent shared with us how they created a peace-making circle to enable them to move through an issue:

The next session was a peace-making session, for everyone to talk about [the conflict which had arisen]. We did the usual beginning check-in, and then we did a round of the facts of what happened, so everyone had to just talk about the fact, not their personal experiences of what happened from their perspective. Then we did a round of how you felt about what happened – like "I felt really unsafe when that happened" and "I didn't know how to respond." Then we did a round of what you would have needed to make it feel better. So, you know, "I need to know that we're going to keep to the rules we have agreed, or change them together." And then we had a round of resolution, what are our next steps now to make sure that everyone feels okay with it.

3   Pete Walker, *Complex PTSD: From Surviving to Thriving*

4   Resmaa Menakem, *My Grandmother's Hands: Racialized Trauma and the Pathway to Mending our Hearts and Bodies,* has another good blueprint for this which he calls the 5 anchors.

5   Sarah Peyton, *Your Resonant Self: Guided Meditations and Exercises to Engage Your Brain's Capacity for Healing*

You may choose to follow a similar model. In addition, here are some steps we've developed that can help you approach specific conflicts within your Red Tent:

✴ When an issue arises in a Red Tent, particularly if it triggers you personally in any way, take time for yourself to discern what you need. You may need time to process it for yourself, perhaps with support, before you are ready to discuss it with others who are involved. It might be that you need to have a good rant, cry, rage or acknowledge shock and disbelief. This could include: stopping, breathing, moving and allowing what is coming up for you personally (assuming something is). Being present and really feeling it in your body. You might use the process which is described above to settle your system. Think about how you can discharge any strong emotions that you feel in a safe and constructive way and how people in your Tent might be able to help and assist you at this time.

✴ When addressing a problem, consider how you might resolve issues together and perhaps commit to the intention to 'resolve it and grow' through this process. We suggest that you use a held circle to give each woman involved an opportunity to speak and listen. Using a circle for this can help enable a process of connection and honesty.

✴ You might also need to arrange to meet with a person (or group of people) who have highlighted that there is an issue or who you want to raise an issue with separately from a held circle. Plan what you want to say and how you want to say it before you are in conversation. Creating a connection is important so it might be better to have this conversation on the phone or in person rather than by email, message or social media.

✴ Clarify the 'facts'. [6] In other words, begin by getting clear about what you can all agree on, in terms of what happened: just the things that a camera could see. Sometimes this stage may be enough to resolve a conflict that has been caused by people having different 'facts' – in other words a different understanding of an issue.

---

6   This process draws on our own practice as well as Mary Ann's practice as a Shadow Work Coach and Action Learning Facilitator and Aisha's experience as a Trainer in community and volunteer groups on Nonviolent Communication inspired by Marshall Rosenberg

✱ Share feelings. Explain how you personally felt in relation to the 'facts'. Invite the other person or people involved to do the same. At each stage listen with the attention and respect you would like to be heard. Being quiet so someone can speak is essential to give time for what they are saying to really land with you.

✱ Remember you are not responsible for other people's feelings, but you are responsible for your own. In other words, you cannot control how other people react, but you can own your feelings and reactions by slowing down, taking time to sense what you are feeling and name it. Do you feel angry, sad, ashamed? Naming this will help you to *be* with what is coming up. Try not to take what someone says personally but to allow yourself to listen to what they are saying and notice what feelings are arising in you. If it feels difficult, ask someone to help you process it.

✱ You may need to ask an uncomfortable question to open the door to an important conversation. It may feel counter-intuitive, but if you feel discomfort, you can still choose to go towards it, not away. In the early part of this book, we talked about the discomfort many white people feel in having conversations about race. We explained that our ability to avoid it, to not talk about it, is part of what sustains white supremacy. We could say this about other oppressive issues too. Avoiding them is always a choice for the privileged. It's always a choice for someone who is not directly impacted. The more privilege we have, be it cis, white, able-bodied, neuro-normative, heterosexual, middle-classed, reproductive or something else we have not named here, the more we need to *choose* discomfort, recognising that it is not, as we may have been taught, the thing we need to run away from, but rather it may well be an indication of the system arising in us. For example, when white supremacy arises in us and our conditioning tells us it isn't our fault, we are one of the good ones and we don't want to talk about the harm we have caused, we have a choice: we can run away from the discomfort, or we can move towards it and seek to learn its lessons about what is so deeply wrong with our society. This gives us the opportunity to choose to uphold systems of oppression or resist them as they arise within us. All this reflection, of course, can take time. In the moment you may not be able to discern the right path. You may need space to process. You may need time to think. This is where the rush to solve or fix a problem can also be the enemy of change. We don't want to leave problems open forever, but we may need time to process them ourselves before we address them together. Let's practice balancing this, however uncomfortable it might seem.

★ Ask open questions (a question that has a range of possible responses, not just 'yes' or 'no') like, "Please, tell me more so I can understand better."

★ Share what you would each like to see as an outcome and what you are prepared to do to make it possible.

★ Ask yourself what you need to learn or unlearn in order to address this is- sue. We make judgements all the time, but the useful part is to know that you are always speaking to some extent from your own judgement – hold it slightly away from yourself to see it more clearly and be able to reflect.

★ Review a number of approaches to resolving the issue and discuss the potential outcomes and possible alternatives to each one. Agree a way forward or set a time to be in touch again.

Don't underestimate the courage and effort these conversations take for all involved. The alternative is to ignore an issue and pretend it is not there. But feelings left unattended and unaddressed are the shadows that linger in our society causing pain and hurt for everyone. The things we avoid resolving can often grow into larger problems when they are unattended.

As LaSara FireFox Allen helps us see that, "for a structure to be resilient, it must be able to withstand disturbance and still function. For a group process to be resilient, it must be able to take a blow and keep thriving... In order to continue actively evolving, a system must not get stuck. For a structure to evolve it must adapt to new parameters, let go of parts that are no longer working, allow itself to be shaped by past experience and by current need. In order to be responsive, a group must be able to absorb new members and adapt to new input. It must be able to sense, listen, and take appropriate action at the right time."[7]

Even if you feel unequipped to resolve an issue, it does not mean that you can't still set the intention to seek to 'resolve it and grow'. We want to invite you to embrace difficult conversations, even when you have no idea what the outcome will be. We cannot make the map until we have travelled the

---

7   Allen, LaSara FireFox. *Jailbreaking the Goddess: A Radical Revisioning of Feminist Spirituality*

road, and believe us, we are on this path with you and will always be. Learning and unlearning a million times over.

Commitment

I want to be strong enough to change. [...]We are not a fragile people. We are an adaptive, resilient, constantly changing species in a constantly changing world and we are strong enough to change now. This moment requires us to be strong enough to change and willing to change and, dare I say, excited to change. And if you are going to be excited to change, you are going to have to deal with being visionary at times, being wrong at times, the mess of it all.

adrienne maree brown [8]

We can get some bonus points for using words like inclusive and open, but passing around big words is meaningless unless we are prepared to do the work and unlearn what we thought we knew in order to live our intentions. This means that when we want to create community, sustain connection and grow a collective Red Tent we need to decide and commit to having the intention to resolve conflict and grow together. We are in it when things start to wobble, when we are filled with doubt, when something happens that shakes up what we think we know and believe. This commitment to having the intention to 'resolve it and grow' when things are difficult is what community really looks like.

We are each human, we each have our own stories, and when we come together conflict will arise at some point. With this intention you can help it be as generative as possible, accepting that there are some conflicts and disagreements that may become difficult and yes, even impossible, to resolve. At some point we guarantee that there will be a moment when you feel upset, sad or angry. You may feel overwhelmed, unworthy, or like there is no way through. We know, and we have been there countless times, putting our

8 *Finding Our Way* podcast with Prentis Hemphill, "Episode 2 – Visioning with adrienne maree brown"

heart into small things, big projects and innumerable tiny tasks. This is why it is so important that you decide on this side of that moment that you will face any challenge with the intention to resolve conflict and grow through the experience. And yes, eventually you may also need to walk away. We are not suggesting you stay in situations of conflict that are harming you. We are not suggesting that there is always a way. But we are suggesting that we see conflict as generative, and something out of which we can emerge changed, individually and collectively.

You never know, you might find that by unpacking the difficult moment with support from others that you learn new things about yourself. The challenge may bring you closer to people and deepen your understanding of the strength and resilience of women in connection. Community can crack us wide open with everything falling to pieces and then love and connection can also flood in to hold fast and bind together those fragments to make it strong like nothing else. It is too beautiful to miss.

12.

CLOSING A RED TENT

Sometimes Red Tents close. Just as we see conflict as something that can be generative, so we see things closing – one door shutting – as something we can choose to embrace. Closing one chapter can be the most important step in creating the space and opening for something new. Nothing, not our lives, nor our planet, have been built to last forever.

And so sometimes we can choose to let go of our shared spaces with joy and gratitude. We invite you to do so consciously and make arrangements to bring things to a close, involving as many in the community in this ending as you can. This may involve giving some time to bring it to an end and having a closing circle that acknowledges the end and what has led to this being a time to close.

Other times, we might choose to step away personally and, if our community structure is strong, to hand the Red Tent space over to another group of women. There might be many reasons we choose to step away, we might be moving, or a new phase might be beginning in our lives, but again we can create ways to honour these transitions, to say farewell, to hand over with blessing.

In Brighton each of us who was involved in starting the Red Tent has had periods of stepping back to have a baby, go travelling or because work contracts took us out of the city for a time. Some of us have started new things that have met a different need or deepened our practice of meeting in community and taken it in a new direction. This happened over a number of years as we dropped away and other women stepped up. For my part I had taken a period of time away to live abroad but always returned and was welcomed back to my place in holding the community. In the end I moved away for good with a small baby and a head and heart full of new plans.

Each of us founders has our own stories, but because we stepped out gradually, the Red Tent has managed to continue with new women reshaping it to meet and adapt to new ways of doing things. It was not always an easy transition and some carried the community on weary shoulders for a while to make sure it really would survive and thrive after we all stepped back. But incredibly it did and is in a new cycle of change.

Aisha

Check-out

When we close our Red Tents, we invite women to *check-out*. To do this we gather together again, in a circle, like we did at the beginning of our time together and we share something to help us leave the space and to feel complete. If you have had a way of checking in that travelled clockwise around the circle passing to each woman's left, you may want to reverse this for the check-out and go anti-clockwise. This helps to embody a sense of weaving together and then unravelling at the end.

Sometimes time is short and so this doesn't last long. The closing ritual could be as simple as: "To close the circle let's blow out the candles together!"

Other times we might allow more time for this, so that there is space for thoughts and reflections to be shared.

Usually we invite women to go round in a circle again and share something, perhaps a brief reflection on their experience of the Red Tent that day or something else that they are taking away with them.

We think it's important to end well, and so in that spirit we also wanted to end this book with a check-out of sorts too.

Aisha Checking Out

I'm Aisha. I have always been someone who has doubted everything that is mainstream and popular. Somehow, if everyone loves it, then maybe I won't. I think we all find ways to 'other' ourselves, to sit on the doormat and never by the fire. The thing about a Red Tent is that it provides an opportunity for everyone to warm their feet by the embers. It can be a brave space in which to heal from the patriarchy, a place that acknowledges the trauma of systemic racism, and which disrupts the binary world that is oppressive and limiting. It has the potential to be something found in multiple communities the world over. That excites me. That makes me feel connected to the idea of a place that fosters a sense of belonging as paramount. That kind of popular I can get with.

Sitting in the slow pace of a circle has made me a better person. I'm able to listen – properly listen – to other people. It's helped me accept people as they are and in doing so, myself. I'm able to hold space for emotion, the really big kinds and the subtle too. Without a doubt that makes me a more relaxed parent. I don't fix every friction, I hold back and let it all be there in a messy jumble. Having so many women around me as inspiration means I feel a little less alone, less confused, less divided: relief that I don't need to live it all myself. I can make sense of more pieces, shared pieces from others, that shape my vision.

I have told my tales, the fragments of thoughts that start in the dark and end up clearer and lighter. Moving my mouth, hearing my voice and making sense of things I didn't know I felt. In short, I am here because you are here. I need you and you can need me. Whether the sun is out or not, we may as well rest a moment, speak a little, and feel our edges as we take in the rays.

Red Tents provide a place of refuge for me to heal from the damage of toxic oppression within society. It builds me up on the inside, helping to reform the places in me that have been devalued, rejected or abandoned. It makes me see the worth of my own story, my own experiences. It allows me to rest just for a short while in a place that feels like a temporary home, where I can breathe. I start to belong in groups of people rather than simply striving to fit. No longer needing to adapt and round some edges to conform and be liked.

As I learn about deep rest and try to meet myself in that place, I want to know what we will rise for as much as what we will rest from. I hope you join us in creating resilient community, whether it is a Red Tent or something similar. For me, being radical with our collective care, unlearning the division that causes us all harm and creating liberatory spaces that reimagine our world is critical right now. Let's give it energy, give it time, give it a whole lot of ourselves and take what we need. Let the mutual connections ripple over into all aspects of our lives, so that we have the strength to question power, disrupt stereotypes and offer different ways of being that bring change.

Writing this book through a difficult pregnancy and post-natal depression has been the backdrop for me. Literally being at my limits while reflecting on how many people are barely getting through each day has felt like a place of connection. A place of hope where I could use my voice and disrupt my silence. That hope, this hope, the hope I have, now passes to you.

Mary Ann Checking Out

Writing this book has been a process, but I feel like we did what we came for. And that feels good. I hope you'll take an idea that you can plant as a seed and grow in your own way.

I imagine gatherings sprouting all over the place. In kitchens. In halls. In work-spaces and online. I imagine women not only resting and caring for each other, but increasingly also resisting the systems that divide and seek to destroy us.

I hope we've encouraged you to want to develop an anti-racist practice. To root into your own practices. To honour what has been taught to you. To create your own rituals...but not to erase where you learnt from. Hold it all with reverence. Find a part of you that remembers – through your genes, long long before your birth or any known genealogy – what it might have felt like to be without white supremacy and root into the possibility that the world could be without it again.

I know this book is one in millions of things that might contribute to the fall of all that is wrong with our current culture. I know it's hard to weave together the bits we can do and be responsible for, and the big mess of the political problems of this world we have inherited. Sometimes it feels like we will never overcome them.

But I do choose to see these as times when anything is possible. And so, whilst there is much to fear and feel anger about right now, I also carry some grains of hope.

We can't see where we are on the long arc of human life on this planet in our limited spans of time here. But I choose to believe it might be possible to play a small part in the dismantling of individualistic, oppressive, racist, capitalist and patriarchal systems.

And that's the spirit in which we offer this book.

I've been reading some of my grandmother's writing. Radical talk about sex for the 1960s and 70s that feels so very dated in many ways to me now. But I see her spirit in me and in this book. A spirit that would not countenance being silent about things that so deeply affect us. A spirit that dared to challenge the wisdom of her day.

In the arc of history, the evidence is that change not only happens, it's a certainty.

Perhaps our only choice is how to play our own small part in directing its flow.

For me Red Tents can be a vehicle that helps us be open to change, to welcome rather than resist it. To build in ourselves a part that's like, "I know I'm imperfect, and that shit things have happened to me and been done by me and yet I am here to embrace change, to welcome accountability, to dare to grow."

It's less about this book being a mark in the sand and more about it gently helping direct one tiny part of a vast river.

I don't know for sure if, like Ben Okri wrote, "Our future is greater than our past"[9] but I don't want to keep on playing a part in maintaining a status quo that is destroying us.

And so, I check out with grains of hope. That those who read this book may see in it some threads they can grab hold of and weave change with.

Maybe with some of what we have shared here new Red Tents will start, people will meet in new ways to create community.

Maybe things will grow out of this that I can't imagine right now.

Call it a Red Tent. Call it something else. But build collective ways to meet these moments. Cherish one another and let yourself be in the midst of change.

The willingness to welcome transformation is something we must build together. Urgently.

And finally, I know for sure that in a few years, if not sooner, we will see all the gaps in what we have written here.

May you forgive the imperfections in what you have read, take what you like and leave the rest. Make what's useful your own, and soar with it towards a world filled with liberation and care.

9   Ben Okri, *Mental Fight: An Anti-Spell for the 21st Century*

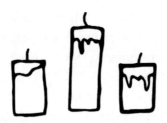

OUR THANKS

This book is nothing if it is not collective work. We want to thank all of the people who generously spoke to us and whose voices are woven through this book as well as all the women we are both in community with in this work on the Red Tent Directory and through Women in Power in the UK. We especially want to thank ALisa Starkweather for introducing the idea of Red Tents to us, for writing our Foreword and inspiring us in this work.

Abi, Agnes, Ali, Ali W, Alexandra, Amy, Anashee, Andrea, Angela, Angie, Aneta, Anna, Barbara, Beth, Becca, Bera, Cali, Camille, Carla, Carly, Cathy, Clare, Clare, Claire, Debbie, Elaine, Emily, Emma, Eva, Gabriella, Heidi, Heidi Hinda, Jane, Jenn, Jessica, Jess, Jill, Jo, Jodi, Julia, Juliet, Karen, Karen, Kaaren, Katrina, Kerstin, Kesty, Kim, Kit, Kristina, Lara, Leigh-Anne, Lily, Lu, Loose, Lou, Mads, Madeleine, Mandy, Margot, Martina, Melonie, Michelle, Natalie, Nicola, Olivia, Olivia, Pascale, Pauline, Persia, Rachael, Reana, Rebecca, Renée, Ruby, Sal, Sama, Sandhya, Sanita, Sophie, Steph, Su, Susannah, Susan, Susana, Tamara, Tasha, Tessa, Vanessa, Vanessa, Yanick, Zoe and Zoë Le Fay.

They come from far and wide including:

Abergavenny, Aegina, Amsterdam, Austin, Aylsham, Basel, Bedfordshire, Berkhamsted, Birmingham, Brighton, Brussels, Bucharest, Budapest, Caerphilly, Cardiff, Caversham, Cilgerran, Cork, Copenhagen, Cumbria, Curico, Edinburgh, Exmoor, Gwynedd, Hayle, Herdecke, Hitchin & Letchworth Garden City, Isle of Arran, Istanbul, Leamington Spa, Leeds, Leon, Liverpool, London, Lyon, Maidenhead, Maenclochog, Manchester, Manitoba, New Forest, Oslo, Paris, Penzance, Plymouth, Richmond, Salisbury, Sevenoaks, Sheffield, Sevenoaks, Sicily, Sintra, St Albans, Stroud, Swansea, Switzerland, Thorpe Morieux, Toronto, Wakefield and West Sussex.

We want to especially honour and remember Mandy, who held a vibrant vision for her Red Tent in Cornwall and sadly did not live to see this book published.

We are also grateful to Lorie, Madhu, Marxe, Fiona, Teresa, Vanessa, Joan, Louise, Yeshe and Lucy for their input on the Womancraft side.

From Aisha

This book has been a wild ride constantly shifting and shaping under our fingers. It has been the deepest honour to write it with you, Mary Ann, and share an insight into how your beautiful mind works. There is simply no way I could have done anything like this alone. We have had simultaneous breakthroughs and breakdowns that have pushed this book into being a more honest depiction of the things that are most precious to us. It's a rare blessing to find someone whose rants and revelations reflect your own. I never want to stop learning alongside you.

Thank you to my mum for teaching me how to really listen and for reminding me how strong I am. To Pauline and Jerry for showing me what it feels like to be welcomed into a loving home – it has enabled me to do the same for others. Thanks to my sister Rachel for reminding me that all you need to do is plant seeds if you want flowers. I am grateful to my brother John for long discussions that expand my horizon. And for the sharp wit of my sisters in life Claire, Emma and Zoe who help me see sense.

Throwing petals at the feet of my original Red Tent sisters: Elaine, Jill, Becca and Adi. I am the person I am because of our wide and deep discussions and what we created. This book is a tribute to all we learnt together.

Deepest gratitude to all the women who have been involved in this book and the many generous women who have helped with the Red Tent Directory, especially our current team. You make it all a pleasure. And Lucy, Leigh and Patrick at Womancraft Publishing thank you for believing in the initial sparks of this project. We've come a long way because of you.

In this world, I've found friends who have unearthed parts of myself I didn't know I had. Here's to the ravers, the mamas, the cunt council collective, the rainbow miles, the wild women, the sweet pea grower, the Llantwit beach treasures and to my oldest friend who always makes the sun come out. And to Colette, thank you for sharing your love. We are still sharing it for you.

Thank you to all the women who lived before me, I think I've inherited your determination and hopefully some of your humour. And Barnaby who joins me in this orbit around the sun. My love for you exploded into my life. You taught me how to be silent and look at the sky. Thank you to Stella for showing me how to play; I delight in watching you grow. And to my smiling son, Louis, who grew in my belly, was birthed and breastfed throughout the journey of writing this book.

From Mary Ann

Deep gratitude to Aisha, this book is not just the work of these two years but truly of the ten years we have been connected. In many ways, we have a working relationship like no other and I really am not sure I could have co-authored a book like this with anyone else. Endless gratitude to you and for all that you are. Deep thanks to Mads for causing us to meet and to Jo for setting me off on a journey that led to a much-needed change in my life and towards our meeting.

To Nicola and Karen for hosting Red Tents in your homes where I began to learn what it meant to truly rest in the company of other women and to so, so many other women spread across all this earth's continents – too many to mention each by name – whose friendship and sisterhood I have learnt to value deeply. I feel deeply grateful to be living at a time in which connection and interdependence across borders is not only technically possible but my lived reality, especially in these pandemic times.

Rachel, you have been with the ancestors for many years now, but I remain grateful always for a friendship that offered me the first inkling that the liberating connection between women, which we speak about in this book, might be possible. It was also you with whom I first shared writing, in much the same way this book has been written, sharing our individual thoughts with one another, woman to woman, and then weaving them together in this book.

To Hannah, my blood sister. You were the first woman whom I felt sisterhood and shared experience with and to my parents, Jean and Dudley for birthing me and creating in me a questioning and liberatory mindset. To my grandparents Eveline Joan, Margot, Francis and Ted, and all my ancestors for living through more difficult times and still dreaming me into being.

And last but not least to Edward and Matthew. Matthew without you I could not and would not have written this. Endless gratitude for the combination of space and sanctuary that is our marriage. I am so, so glad to be moving through these times with you. Edward, over the course of my writing this book you have grown into someone who is able to both encourage me in my writing and to read it for yourself. It's an honour to call myself your Mum.

RESOURCES

Find the nearest Red Tent to you on our global Red Tent listing site the Red Tent Directory: redtentdirectory.com

A transgender welcome logo for Red Tents can be found here: barefootheartsong.blogspot.com/2019/10/welcome-women-all.html. Please follow the instructions if you would like to use it.

The following is a collection of resources that have inspired us, or that we have quoted from in this book. We recommend exploring them, but including a book here does not mean that we endorse everything that they say. It does mean that their ideas or concepts are relevant to some of what we write about in this book and that we want to credit them and invite you to dive deeper into their work. Where we have quoted directly we have also referenced the ideas we draw on throughout the book.

Books

Agarwal, Pragya. *Sway: Unravelling Unconscious Bias*

Akala, Natives. *Race and Class in the Ruins of Empire*

Allen, LaSara FireFox. *Jailbreaking the Goddess: A Radical Revisioning of Feminist Spirituality*

Allione, Tsultrim. *Feeding your Demons: Ancient Wisdom for Resolving Inner Conflict*

Baldwin, Christina. *Calling the Circle: The First and Future Culture*

Bates, Laura. *Men Who Hate Women: From Incels to Pickup Artists, the Truth about Extreme Misogyny and How it Affects Us All*

brown, adrienne maree. *Emergent Strategy: Shaping Change, Changing Worlds* brown, adrienne maree. *Pleasure Activism: The Politics of Feeling Good*

brown, adrienne maree. *We Will Not Cancel Us – And Other Dreams of Transformative Justice*

Carrellas, Barbara. *Urban Tantra: Second Edition: Sacred Sex for the Twenty-First Century*

Chown, Vicky and Walker Kim. *The Handmade Apothecary: Healing Herbal Remedies*

Chown, Vicky and Walker Kim. *The Herbal Remedy Handbook: Treat Everyday Ailments Naturally, from Coughs and Colds to Anxiety and Eczema*

Clark-Coates, Zoe. *Saying Goodbye: A Personal Story of Baby Loss and 90 Days of Support to Walk You Through Grief*

Cooper, Clare. *Milestones of Motherhood*

Dabiri, Emma. *Don't Touch My Hair*

Diamant, Anita. *The Red Tent*

Duerk, Judith. *I Sit Listening to the Wind: Woman's Encounter Within Herself*

Duerk, Judith. *Circle of Stones: Woman's Journey To Her Self*

Eddo-Lodge, Reni. *Why I'm No Longer Talking to White People About Race*

Ensler, Eve. *The Vagina Monologues*

Estes, Clarissa Pinkola. *Women Who Run with the Wolves: Contacting the Power of the Wild Woman*

Feldman, Christina. *The Quest of the Warrior Woman: Women as Mystics, Healers and Guides*

Gbowee, Leymah. *Mighty Be Our Powers: How Sisterhood, Prayer, and Sex Changed a Nation at War*

George, Demetra. *Mysteries of the Dark Moon: The Healing Power of the Dark Goddess*

Goldsmith, Esuantsiwa Jane. *The Space Between Black and White*

Hedley, Christopher and Shaw, Non. *A Herbal Book of Making and Taking*

Hill, Maisie. *Period Power: Harness Your Hormones and Get Your Cycle Working for You*

Heginworth, Ian Siddons. *Environmental Arts Therapy and the Tree of Life*

Kaba, Mariame and Hassan, Shira. *Fumbling Towards Repair: A Workbook for Community Accountability Facilitators*

Kenton, Leslie. *Passage to Power: Natural Menopause Revolution*

Kindred, Glennie. *Sacred Earth Celebrations*

Kindred, Glennie and Garner, Lu. *Creating Ceremony*

Kimmerer, Robin Wall. *Braiding Sweetgrass: Indigenous Wisdom, Scientific Knowledge and the Teaching of Plants*

Khan-Cullors, Patrisse, and Bandele, Asha. *When They Call You a Terrorist: A Black Lives Matter Memoir*

Kwakye, Chelsea and Ogunbiyi, Ore. *Taking Up Space: The Black Girl's Manifesto for Change*

Leidenfrost, Isadora, PhD and Starkweather, ALisa. *The Red Tent Movement: A Historical Perspective*

Levine, Peter. A. *Waking the Tiger: Healing Trauma*

Lister, Lisa. *Code Red: Know Your Flow, Unlock Your Superpowers, and Create a Bloody Amazing Life. Period*

Lorde, Audre. *A Burst of Light: and Other Essays*

Maathai, Wangari. *Unbowed: My Autobiography*

Maddox, Rachael. *Secret Bad Girl: A Sexual Trauma Memoir and Resolution Guide*

Mahoney, Mary and Mitchell, Lauren. *The Doulas: Radical Care for Pregnant People*

Magdalena, Yarrow. *Rituals – Simple & Radical Practices for Enchantment in Times of Crisis*

Menakem, Resmaa. *My Grandmother's Hands: Racialized Trauma and the Pathway to Mending Our Hearts and Bodies*

Meulenbelt, A, Leenhouts, J, Bijman, S and van Manen, B. *For Ourselves – Our Bodies and Sexuality – from a Woman's Point of View*

Nicholas, Chani. *You Were Born for This: Astrology for Radical Self-Acceptance*

Okri, Ben. *Mental Fight: An Anti-Spell for the 21st Century*

Owens, Lama Rod. *Love and Rage: The Path of Liberation through Anger*

Peacock, Jardana. *Practice Showing Up: A Guidebook for White People Working for Racial Justice*

Pearce, Lucy. H. *Full Circle Health: Integrated Health Charting for Women*

Pearce, Lucy. H. *Moon Time: Harness the Ever-Changing Energy of Your Menstrual Cycle*

Pearce, Lucy. H. *Reaching for the Moon – A Girl's Guide to her Cycles*

Perry, Grayson. *The Descent of Man*

Peyton, Sarah. *Your Resonant Self: Guided Meditations and Exercises to Engage Your Brain's Capacity for Healing*

Phipps, Alison. *Me, Not You: The Trouble with Mainstream Feminism*

Piepzna-Samarasinha, Leah Lakshmi and Dixon, Ejeris. *Beyond Survival: Strategies and Stories from the Transformative Justice Movement*

Piepzna-Samarasinha, Leah Lakshmi. *Care Work: Dreaming Disability Justice*

Pope, Alexandra and Wurlitzer, Sjanie Hugo. *Wild Power: Discover the Magic of Your Menstrual Cycle and Awaken the Feminine Path to Power*

Remer, Molly. *Restoring Women to Ceremony: The Red Tent Resource Kit*

Renée Taylor, Sonya. *The Body Is Not an Apology: The Power of Radical Self-Love*

Rosenberg, Marshall B. *Non-Violent Communication: A Language of Life. Create your Life, Your Relationships, and our World in Harmony with Your Values.* 2nd Edition

Rothschild, Liz. *Outside the Box: Everyday Stories of Death, Bereavement and Life*

Rothschild, Marianne. *Dancing with the Rhythms of Life: A Holistic Doctor's Guide for Women*

Russo, Ann. *Feminist Accountability: Disrupting Violence and Transforming Power*

Saad, Layla F. *Me and White Supremacy: How to Recognise Your Privilege, Combat Racism and Change the World*

Serano, Julia. *Whipping Girl: A Transsexual Woman on Sexism and the Scapegoating of Femininity*

Serano, Julia. *Excluded: Making Feminist and Queer Movements More Inclusive*

Sfez, Camille. *La Puissance du Feminine*

Turner, Toko-pa. *Belonging: Remembering Ourselves Home*

van der Kolk, Bessel. *The Body Keeps the Score: Mind, Brain and Body in the Transformation of Trauma*

Villanueva, Edgar. *Decolonizing Wealth*

Walker, Alice. *In Search of Our Mother's Gardens*

Walker, Pete. *Complex PTSD: From Surviving to Thriving*

Wilding, Amy Bammel. *Wild & Wise: Sacred Feminine Meditations for Women's Circles*

Williams, Angel Kyodo and Owens, Rod. *Radical Dharma Talking Race, Love, and Liberation*

Also, Boston Women's Health Collective. *Our Bodies, Ourselves.* (A number of different versions and revision of this text are available. It was first published in 1973, but is still worth exploring!)

Film and Audio

Disclosure: Trans Lives on Screen. Netflix

Things We Don't Talk About: Women's Stories from the Red Tent. Isadora Gabrielle Leidenfrost, PhD.

The Red Tent. Television miniseries, Lifetime, 2014.

Adichie, Chimamanda Ngozi, "The Danger of a Single Story", TED. youtube.com/watch?v=D9Ihs241zeg

Mint Faery, "Cleansing Tools for Every Witch: Alternatives to Using Smudge Wands" youtube.com/watch?v=OmVIpEZ0-Ys&t=294

Finding our Way podcast. Prentice Hemphill

Online References

Selected Proceedings from the 2003 Annual Conference of the International Leadership Association, November 6-8, Guadalajara, Jalisco, Mexico ila-net.org/Publications/Proceedings/2003/mgrace.pdf

Adaway Desiree and Fish, Jessica, *Diversity & Inclusion Primer* 2018 adawaygroup.com

Castro, M. "Introducing the Red Tent: A discursive and Critically Hopeful Exploration of Women's Circles in a Neoliberal Postfeminist Context." (2020), *Sociological Research Online*. ISSN 1360-7804

Chigudu, Hope and Chigudu, Rudo. "Strategies for Building an Organisation with Soul." airforafrica.org/wp-content/uploads/2015/09/Strategies-for-Building-an-Organisation-with-Soul-for-web1.pdf

Clements, Mary Ann. "How we Treat Ourselves." how-matters.org/2017/06/21/how-we-treat-ourselves

Clements, Mary Ann. "What capacities might we, as white people in international development, need to build in ourselves in order to commit to anti-racist practice?" medium.com/@maryannmhina/what-capacities-might-we-as-white-people-in-international-development-need-to-build-in-ourselves-49e765a3151b

Clements, Mary Ann. "What Role Can Privileged White People Play in International Development?" brightthemag.com/white-supremacy-race-ngo-what-role-can-white-privilege-people-play-international-development-3c648c7252e9

Clements, Mary Ann. "Resisting the commoditisation of self-care and building our capacity for collective care." medium.com/@maryannmhina/resisting-the-commoditisation-of-self-care-building-our-capacity-for-collective-care-b8307deddea1

Horn, Jessica. "Decolonising emotional well-being and mental health in development." *African feminist innovations in Gender and Development Journal* vol 28. Issue 1 Edited by Clements. Mary Ann & Sweetman, Caroline. policy-practice.oxfam.org.uk/publications/decolonising-emotional-well-being-and-mental-health-in-development-african-femi-620960

Johnson, Maisha Z. "What's Wrong with Cultural Appropriation? These 9 Answers Reveal its Harm"

LadyBeard Magazine – especially The Mind Issue – ladybeardmagazine.co.uk/shop/the-mind-issue

McClure, Tess. "Dark Crystals: the brutal reality behind a booming wellness craze." theguardian.com/lifeandstyle/2019/sep/17/healing-crystals-wellness-mining-madagascar

Nolan, Colette. "Cunt owners are not always women" cherishthecunt. wordpress.com/2014/07/08/cunt-owners-are-not-always-women/

Raimondi, Gwynn. "These times do not have to be traumatic" medium. com/@gwynnraimondi/these-times-do-not-have-to-be-traumatic-1eeda284bd89

Olorenshaw, Vanessa. "The Red Tent Movement and a Circle of Women" huffingtonpost.co.uk/vanessa-olorenshaw/the-red-tent-movement_b_8091348.html

Payne, Kendra. "A Black Herbalist these are my 3 Favorite Herbalism Books" theherbalacademy.com/black-herbalism-books/

Piepzna-Samarasinha, Leah Lakshmi. "Fragrance Free and Scent Free Guidelines." brownstargirl.org/fragrance-free-femme-of-colour-genius/

Power, Camilla. "Did Gender Egalitarianism Make Us Human? Or, If Graeber And Wengrow Won't Talk About Sex…" youtube.com/watch?v=xr_7qbI0Gbk

Saad, Layla F. "I need to talk to spiritual white women about white supremacy (Part One)" laylafsaad.com/poetry-prose/white-women-white-supremacy-1

Scheepers, Ella and Lakhani, Ishtar. "Caution! Feminists at work: building organizations from the inside out." From *Gender and Development,* Vol 28, no1, Reimagining International Development, Edited by Mary Ann Clements and Caroline Sweetman

Sequoia, Lily. *She Who Knows* magazine, May 2018. "Obituary. Activist, Artist, Poet, Writer, Educator, Mother. Colette Joan Nolan 17.11.1982 – 13.02.2018" inkdistribution.co.uk/magazines/she-who-knows/

Solnit, Rebecca. "Trans women pose no threat to cis women, but we pose a threat to them if we make them outcasts" theguardian.com/commentisfree/2020/aug/10/trans-rights-feminist-letter-rebecca-solnit,

VeneKlasen, Lisa. "Last Word – How Does Change Happen?" (2006) *Development,* 49, (155–161) justassociates.org/sites/justassociates.org/files/development_journal.veneklasen_0.pdf

"Mayer-Rokitansky-Küster-Hauser Syndrome". Rare Diseases.org rarediseases. org/rare-diseases/mayer-rokitansky-kuster-hauser-syndrome/

"Witchcraft", UK Parliament. parliament.uk/about/living-heritage/ transformingsociety/private-lives/religion/overview/witchcraft/

Podcasts

Macklin, Sophie. "Practicising Collective Grief." Episode 57. *Change Making Women* changemakingwomen.com/57-practicing-collective-grief-with-sophie-macklin/

Finding Our Way with Prentis Hemphill, (especially Episode 2 – "Visioning" with adrienne maree brown)

Herbalists without Borders hwbglobal.org/herbal-action-podcast.html

How to Survive the End of the World endoftheworldshow.org

On Being with Krista Tippett (especially onbeing.org/programs/resmaa-menakem-notice-the-rage-notice-the-silence/)

Remember who Made Them rememberwhomadethem.com

For the Wild: Episode 102 – "On Decolonizing Birth" forthewild.world/ listen/roots-of-labor-birth-collective-on-decolonizing-birth102

Some of the Campaigns We Support at the Red Tent Directory

Bloody Good Period: bloodygoodperiod.com – helps asylum seekers access period products.

FRIDA | Young Feminist Fund: youngfeministfund.org – participatory fund supporting young feminist organising around the world.

WEN, Women's Environmental Network Environmenstrual Campaign: wen.org.uk/our-work/environmenstrual/ – campaigns for plastic free and a campaign to raïse awareness of hidden plastic and chemicals in conventional menstrual products and promote reusable and organic options.

Resources and Websites to Explore

Angel Kyodo Williams – angelkyodowilliams.com

The Nap Ministry – instagram.com/thenapministry

Catalyst Project – Anti-Racism for Collective Liberation – collectiveliberation.org

The Circle Way – thecircleway.net

Clare Beloved – clarebeloved.com

Colette Nolan: – Cunt Craft, spoken word and inspiration. cherishthecunt.wordpress.com

Education for Racial Equity Resources – educationforracialequity.com/resources

Elaine Rose Leela – mindfulmenstrualcycle.com

Gwynn Raimondi – gwynnraimondi.com

Healing Solidarity – healingsolidarity.org

Dr Jennifer Mullan – drjennifermullan.com

Karine Bell – karinebell.com/ (includes dedicated resources around trauma and healing for Black women as well as multiracial offerings)

Mary Ann Clements – maryannclements.com

MRKH – mrkh.org.uk

Red Tent Doulas – redtentdoulas.co.uk

Red Tent Temple Movement – redtenttemplemovement.com

Safe Spaces for Black Women – safespacesforblackwomen.com

Shadow Work – shadowwork.eu

Sophie Macklin – instagram.com/sophieamacklin

Women in Power UK – womeninpoweruk.com

Cards

Dear Sister Cards by Desiree Adaway that explore liberatory practice to use in Red Tent Spaces thegamecrafter.com/designers/desiree-adaway

Diverse Tarot Decks and other resources: littleredtarot.com

GLOSSARY OF TERMS

Anti-Racism

A belief in the need to end racism, for people to be treated equally regardless of the colour of their skin and the activism motivated by seeking to end racism.

Capitalism

A system in which the accumulation of capital, profit and other kinds of monetary wealth, takes precedence in the organising of human life.

Equity/Equality

Equity is focused on giving everyone the same chance of achieving or accessing something whereas equality is focused on creating a level playing field for all.

Feminism

A belief in the equality of sexes and of genders and the activism motivated by seeking to make this equity a reality in the world.

Herstory

A history viewed from a female or specifically feminist perspective.

Implicit or Unconscious Bias

Things that we are biased about without our conscious awareness leading us to have thoughts and take actions that give preference to, or remove preference from a specific group, or identity. This is different in character to bias which we enact consciously such as overt forms of racism or sexism.

Patriarchy
A system in which the male and patrilineal take precedent.

Racism
The treatment of people differently based on their so called 'race' or ethnicity and the incorrect inference that that makes them biologically different giving them different traits and/or abilities. Most often based on how they look and the colour of their skin.

Trauma
The response to an event, series of events or long-term experience of society that is deeply distressing and which we are unable to fully process at the time. Our systems respond in a way designed to save us but not to fully integrate what has happened or is happening and/or events of this type which happened to our ancestors and they have not been fully able to process and therefore is passed to us through our DNA.

White Supremacy
A system, evident in human life since at least the 1400s (Villanueva, E. *Decolonizing Wealth*, 2018), in which white bodies are always superior and which has been used as justification for colonialisation, slavery, exploitation and genocide.

ABOUT THE AUTHORS

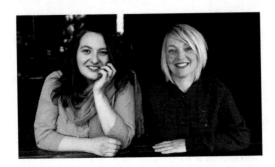

Aisha Hannibal has worked for over twenty years in the charity sector from working in front-line services with people experiencing domestic violence to training teachers in intercultural learning in schools. Creating resilient communities has been an essential part of her work. She learnt a lot about leadership by being a trustee for seven years for an NGO supporting campaigns led by conservation organisations in Russia and Eastern Europe as well as being involved in housing cooperatives in the UK. As a campaigner she set up international projects to educate and empower global and active citizens to promote peace through cross cultural reflection. She currently supports people to establish grassroots groups in the UK to make cities and towns more accessible for walking and cycling. Her commitment to work with women threads through all of her ventures including managing the website for Women in Power UK which runs an initiation programme for women. Her passion for sustainable networks of support underpins her dedication to the Red Tent Directory which she co-founded with Mary Ann 8 years ago.

Mary Ann Clements is a Feminist Writer, Facilitator, Activist and Coach. She worked with Aisha to launch the Red Tent Directory in 2012 and they have run it together since. She believes in the power for women's circles and community to help create change in our world. Mary Ann helps people and organisations explore how the injustice they stand against shows up in them. In so doing she helps them create more space to be part of imagining a radically different future. *Healing Solidarity*, an online annual conference and hub that she initiated, and now runs it together with a multi-racial Advisory Circle, has engaged well over 3000 people in conversations about re-imagining international development and addressing racism within it since 2018. It builds on her two decades experience in the sector, including seven years as the Director of an INGO. She takes an intersectional feminist approach to all her work which has had a particular focus on disability, mental health and women's rights. She is also a Shadow Work Coach, Action Learning Facilitator, TedX Speaker and Movement Practitioner. She's co-host of the podcast, *Change Making Women* and is active in the Women in Power UK Community. She also has many years' experience as a Board Member including as Chair of a Women's Refuge in South London.

ABOUT THE ARTIST

Leigh Millar has always enjoyed dabbling in different arts and crafts from painting and drawing to sewing and felting. In recent years she has found a love for the simple delicacy of handmade papercut designs.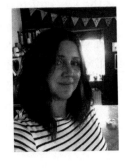

Self-taught, Leigh has run papercutting workshops and takes commissions for her work. She is a mum of three living in a little cottage by the sea in the south of Ireland.

ABOUT WOMANCRAFT

Womancraft Publishing was founded on the revolutionary vision that women and words can change the world. We act as midwife to transformational women's words that have the power to challenge, inspire, heal and speak to the silenced aspects of ourselves.
 We believe that:

✴ books are a fabulous way of transmitting powerful transformation,

✴ values should be juicy actions, lived out,

✴ ethical business is a key way to contribute to conscious change.

 At the heart of our Womancraft philosophy is fairness and integrity. Creatives and women have always been underpaid. Not on our watch! We split royalties 50:50 with our authors. We work on a full circle model of giving and receiving: reaching backwards, supporting TreeSisters' reforestation projects, and forwards via Worldreader, providing books at no cost to education projects for girls and women.
 We are proud that Womancraft is walking its talk and engaging so many women each year via our books and online. Join the revolution! Sign up to the mailing list at womancraftpublishing.com and find us on social media for exclusive offers:

(f) womancraftpublishing

(y) womancraftbooks

(o) womancraft_publishing

Signed copies of all titles available from
shop.womancraftpublishing.com

Wild & Wise: sacred feminine meditations for women's circles and personal awakening

Amy Wilding

The stunning debut by Amy Wilding is not merely a collection of guided meditations, but a potent tool for personal and global transformation. The meditations beckon you to explore the powerful realm of symbolism and archetypes, inviting you to access your wild and wise inner knowing.

Suitable for reflective reading or to facilitate healing and empowerment for women who gather in red tents, moon lodges, women's circles and ceremonies.

This rich resource is an answer to "what can we do to go deeper?" that many in circles want to know.

Jean Shinoda Bolen, MD

Burning Woman

Lucy H. Pearce

2017 Nautilus Award Winner in the program's 'Women' category of books for and about Women's journey. A breath-taking and controversial woman's journey through history – personal and cultural – on a quest to find and free her own power.

Uncompromising and all-encompassing, Pearce uncovers the archetype of the Burning Women of days gone by – Joan of Arc and the witch trials, through to the way women are burned today in cyber bullying, acid attacks, shaming and burnout, fearlessly examining the roots of Feminine power – what it is, how it has been controlled, and why it needs to be unleashed on the world in our modern Burning Times.

A must-read for all women! A life-changing book that fills the reader with a burning passion and desire for change.

Glennie Kindred, author of *Earth Wisdom*

Moon Time:
harness the ever-changing energy
of your menstrual cycle

Lucy H. Pearce

Hailed as 'life-changing' by women around the world, *Moon Time* shares a fully embodied understanding of the menstrual cycle. Full of practical insight, empowering resources, creative activities and passion, this book will put women back in touch with their body's wisdom.

This book is a wonderful journey of discovery. Lucy not only guides us through the wisdom inherent in our wombs, our cycles and our hearts, but also encourages us to share, express, celebrate and enjoy what it means to be female! A beautiful and inspiring book full of practical information and ideas.

Miranda Gray, author of *Red Moon* and *The Optimized Woman*

Walking with Persephone

Molly Remer

Midlife can be a time of great change – inner and outer: a time of letting go of the old, burnout and disillusionment. But how do we journey through this? And what can we learn in the process? Molly Remer is our personal guide to the unraveling and reweaving required in midlife. She invites you to take a walk with the goddess Persephone, whose story of descent into the underworld has much to teach us.

Walking with Persephone is a story of devotion and renewal that weaves together personal experiences, insights, observations, and reflections with experiences in practical priestessing, family life, and explorations of the natural world. It advocates opening our eyes to the wonder around us, encouraging the reader to both look within themselves for truths about living, but also to the earth, the air, the sky, the animals, and plants.

Part memoir, part poetry, part soul guide, Molly's evocative voice is in the great American tradition of sacred nature writing.

USE OF WOMANCRAFT WORK

Often women contact us asking if and how they may use our work.

We love seeing our work out in the world. We love you sharing our words further. And we ask that you respect our hard work by acknowledging the source of the words.

We are delighted for short quotes from our books – up to 200 words – to be shared as memes or in your own articles or books, provided they are clearly accompanied by the author's name and the book's title.

We are also very happy for the materials in our books to be shared amongst women's communities: to be studied by book groups, discussed in classes, read from in ceremony, quoted on social media…with the following provisos:

✴ If content from the book is shared in written or spoken form, the book's author and title must be referenced clearly.

✴ The only person fully qualified to teach the material from any of our titles is the author of the book itself. There are no accredited teachers of this work. Please do not make claims of this sort.

✴ If you are creating a course devoted to the content of one of our books, its title and author must be clearly acknowledged on all promotional material (posters, websites, social media posts).

✴ The book's cover may be used in promotional materials or social media posts. The cover art is copyright of the artist and has been licensed exclusively for this book. Any element of the book's cover or font may not be used in branding your own marketing materials when teaching the content of the book, or content very similar to the original book.

✴ No more than two double page spreads, or four single pages of any book may be photocopied as teaching materials.

We are delighted to offer a 20% discount of over five copies going to one address. You can order these on our webshop, or email us. If you require further clarification, email us at:

info@womancraftpublishing.com